THE FOOD FALLACY

"How much you eat matters less than what you eat."

Text © Andrew E. Strigner 2008

First published in Great Britain in 2008
by MME&T Publications ISBN 978-0-9558803-1-5

Andrew E. Strigner has asserted his right to be identified as the author of this Work in accordance with the Copyrights, Designs and Patents Act 1988.
All rights reserved under International Copyright Conventions.

No part of this publication may be reproduced, stored in a retrieval system, or transmitted in any form or by any means, electronic, mechanical, photocopying, recording or otherwise with the prior permission of the copyright owner.

Typeset by Anne Hanson
Printed and bound in Great Britain
by MME&T Publications
Chipley Manor
Chipley
Newton Abbot
Devon TQ12 6JW

MME&T's policy is to use papers that are natural, renewable and recyclable products made from wood grown in sustainable forests.

Foreword

The Food Fallacy – Dr. Andrew Strigner

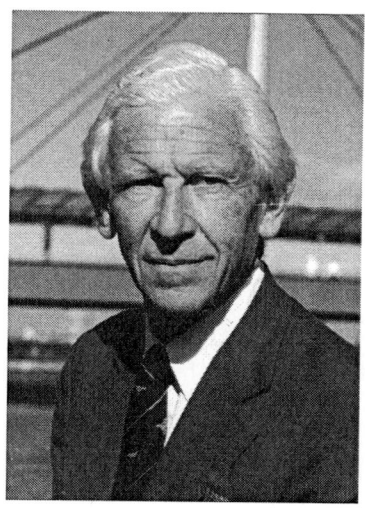

At a time when we are all accustomed to being bombarded with advice on the pros and cons of various foodstuffs and food supplements, claims for therapeutic properties and warnings of health hazards, in the media, in promotional advertisements and in official proclamations, it is a positive joy to peruse these pages of authoritative and comprehensive analysis of nutritional science; set out so clearly, so readably, and with delightful flashes of humour. There is something here for all of us, – doctors, patients, mothers, the young and the old, – interesting, instructive and altogether enjoyable.

Andrew Strigner, WWII soldier, physician, homoeopath and hypnotherapist, traces the Origins of Man, and his progress over tens of thousands of years, from hunter-gatherer to agriculturalist, and there is much that we can learn from his progress.

But for most of us today it is a giant stride from the farmyard to the supermarket via the food technologists and processors, interspersed with periodic announcements from the various health agencies. There are so many of the latter that most of us ignore them altogether: others are slaves to them. This fascinating book deals with all of them, and discusses the role of the vitamins, the minerals and the trace metals which occur in our diet. It examines the effects of cooking methods and cookery utensils, and studies aspects of ill-health that are related to nutrition – diabetes, food allergies, heart problems and cancer.

This is not a book to consign to the library shelf. Put it where you can pick it up and read it at any time e.g. with the cookery books, on the coffee table, – perhaps in the loo. Start reading anywhere and you'll find it hard to put down. I read it from cover to cover in two days, and keep on picking it up and re-reading at random. And label pages for friends.

The book is unique, the way it is set out, the illustrations, the quality and style of the text. I have no words to express adequately my admiration for its author.

Sir John Rawlins KBE FRCP FRAeS
Surgeon Vice-Admiral

The Duchess of York

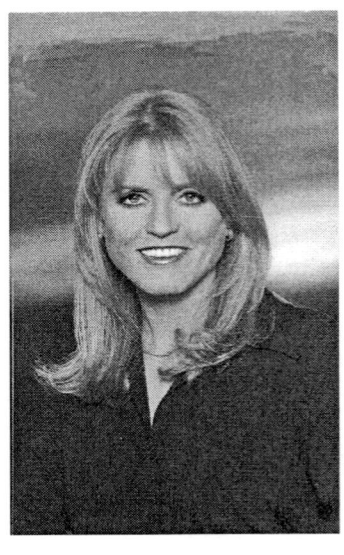

I have known Andrew Strigner for twenty years and am delighted that, at last, he has written this book as I believe that his vast experience and wisdom should be shared.

"The Food Fallacy" is a fascinating book which dispels myths, offers advice and clarifies the basic concept of what constitutes a healthy eating regime. Today, when there are many books on the market regarding health, it is so refreshing to read one which simply advises the reader on how to look after one's body and mind by eating sensibly.

Sarah, Duchess of York

Foreword

I have known Andrew Strigner since I was thirteen years old and forty years later he continues to inspire that awe and confidence that characterises the man. He is a quietly spoken man and a gentle man but above all a gentleman – this is a distinction that only applies to great men and the greatest honour I can do Andrew is to call him a gentleman.

He is a man of immense intelligence and integrity and has identified a huge defect in modern society and that is the dreadful spiral of poor nutrition that has befallen us. Sadly he is not somebody to shout it from the rooftops but his observations are only now coming to general attention. We have only just discovered that although we are surrounded by plenty we are starving from a lack of quality in what we eat. This is reminiscent of the sailor on the ocean where there is "water, water everywhere but not a drop to drink." The difference is that much of our problems is of our own making.

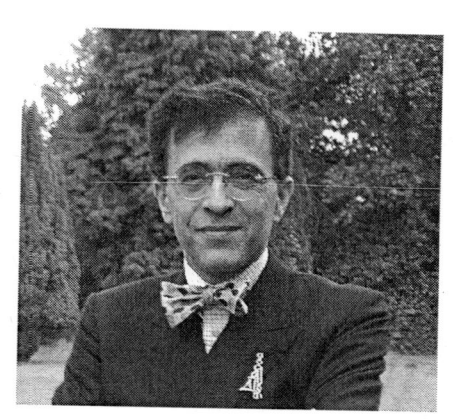

This book is filled with common sense and astute observation and is very concentrated so it bears reading in segments and often, as the messages are clear and intense.

Andrew's experience with nutrition and nutritional needs in relation to general well-being has stood him in great stead over the years and he has been able to salvage patients who have been failed by conventional medicine.

There is nothing alternative, faddist or gimmicky about his advice nor is it driven by the more extreme members of the "nut cutlet" brigade. It is simply common sense and good intelligent advice, those most rare of modern commodities.

One cannot fail to benefit from reading this book and it is a great legacy to a a great man and a great gentleman.

Charles A. Akle BSc MS FRCS.
Consultant Surgeon

The Food Fallacy
Dr. Andrew Strigner 2007

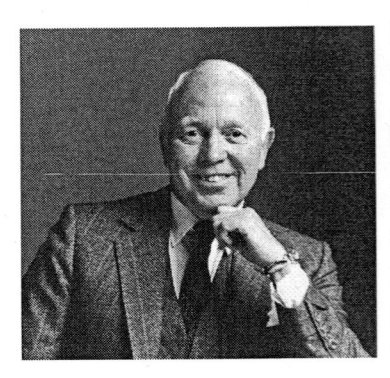

I met Dr. Andrew Strigner in the Summer of 1977. If I had not met him then, I would not be alive today to write this Foreword to *The Food Fallacy*, a book that will feed you for life.

My own life involves a punishing-to-the-body-nine-months-of-the-year global travel schedule in which I am often required to work 18 hours a day.

Simple maintenance is not enough.

The human body is like a Formula One racing car, and equally requires and deserves a similar team of highly trained engineers to make sure that all its operating systems are functioning to their maximum levels, that the fuel (food) is perfect to the last molecule, and that any malfunction can be immediately diagnosed and rapidly corrected.

Having put myself at risk a number of times, I was looking for such a team.

I found the entire team in one man: Dr. Andrew Strigner.

Imagine the qualities you would look for if you had limitless funds and could design the ideal doctor to look after all major aspects of your health from birth to your very senior years, and to write the seminal work on human nutrition. Surely these would include:

- A doctor who knows, intimately, the 'secrets' of nutrition. As a farmer, Dr. Strigner did groundbreaking research on the nutrition of mammals and its effect on their health and behaviours. He was Chairman, now Vice-President, of the McCarrison Society, formed originally by a group of doctors, dentists, veterinarians and others interested in the art and science of nutrition.
- A knowledge of formal Western Scientific Medicine. Dr. Strigner has such qualifications.
- A doctor effective in integrated – not "alternative" – medicine and with an open mind to different cultures and different approaches. Dr. Strigner was Assistant Physician in the Cardiology and Paediatric Departments of the Royal London Homeopathic Hospital. He also has vast knowledge of the histories of nutrition and their effects in all major global communities.

- A doctor who has experience of life outside medicine. Dr. Strigner has been a World War II Army pilot, a traveller, a Martial Artist, a father of three very successful children, and a farmer.
- A doctor held in high esteem by his colleagues and his patients. Dr. Strigner has devoted much of his life to charity work, while simultaneously being the chosen physician to world leaders in many fields. Many, like me, credit him with saving and extending their lives: with being the doyenne of medical nutritionists.
- A doctor who understands and can help you handle the stress of modern life. Dr. Strigner is one the world's leading hypnotherapists.

The book you now hold in your hands is a distillation of over 50 years of work of a giant in the medical field, incorporating Dr. Strigner's vast knowledge from the aforementioned areas. It is the first nutritional work in the modern age that is not a 'prescription' nor a 'diet' nor a 'formula'. It is an objective, witty and caring overview of the entire field of human nutrition. It gives clear and beautifully explained guidelines for how you, as a human being, can nurture yourself.

It is a book that should hold pride of place in the library of every home.

The world has found, in Dr. Strigner, the doctor for whom, and the book for which, it has been searching.

Tony Buzan
Inventor: Mind Maps
Author:
Use Your Head
The Power of Physical Intelligence

The Food Fallacy

Dr. Andrew Strigner 2005

Dr Andrew Strigner is a consultant physician with over 50 years of expertise in clinical medicine and an acknowledged specialist in Nutrition, Hypnosis and Homeopathy.

Graduate of London University, Guy's Hospital and of the Royal London Homeopathic Hospital. Worked at the latter for several years as physician in the paediatric and cardiology departments.

Recognised internationally as an authority on the teaching and clinical use of self-hypnosis, a member of the Medical Hypnosis Association.

Formerly Chairman, presently Vice President of the McCarrison Society for the study of the relationship between Nutrition and Health.

Currently Fellow of the Royal Society of Medicine and The Medical Society of London.

For many years, concurrent with practising medicine, engaged in the breeding and raising of sheep and beef cattle in hill country in the South West of England.

Table of contents

Prefaces	12
Front matter page	13
Introduction	14-17
Chapter 1: **Origin and Evolution**	19-24
Chapter 2: **Agriculture is not natural**	25-36
Chapter 3: **Food**	
– the ancestral diet	39-45
– Adaptation – Survival of the fittest	46-52
– blood groups	47-50
– lectins	51
– tissue types	51
– raw or cooked	52
– latterday culprits: sugar, milk, grains	53-59
Chapter 4: **Food for thought**	
– mental effects	63-66
Chapter 5: **Components of food**	
– Protein	69-71
– Fat, More about Fats, Fats – chemistry	72-79
– Carbohydrates	80 & 81
– Cholesterol	81 & 82
– Fibre	82 & 83
– Water	84 & 85
Chapter 6: **Free Radicals and Antioxidants**	87-93
Chapter 7: **Vitamins** Casimir Funk	97
Preface	99
– A and Beta carotene	100 & 101
– B_1 B_2 B_3 B_5 B_6 B_8 B_9 B_{12}	102 - 107
– C	108
– D	109 & 110
– E	110
– K	111
– Other substances: Inositol	112 & 113
– Choline, Pyrolloquinolone, Ubiquinone and Co Q10,	112
– Betaine and the Homocysteine Cycle	113

Table of contents
continued

Chapter 8: Minerals

–	carbon	117
–	sulphur	117 & 118
–	calcium	118 & 119
–	phosphorus	120
–	magnesium	120 & 121
–	sodium	121 & 122
–	potassium	122
–	chloride (chlorine)	122
–	iron	123
–	zinc	123 & 124
–	chromium	124 & 125
–	copper	125 & 126
–	manganese	126
–	iodine	126 & 127
–	molybdenum	127
–	boron	127
–	cobalt	127 & 128
–	selenium	128 & 129
–	vanadium	129
–	fluoride (fluorine)	130
–	arsenic	130
–	silicon	130
–	bromide (bromine)	130 & 131
–	strontium	131
–	A Miscellany: tin, germanium and nickel	131

Chapter 9: The toxic metals

–	lead	135
–	cadmium	136
–	mercury	136
–	aluminium	137
–	beryllium	137

# Table of contents
continued

Chapter 10:	**Exercise: physical activity**	
	– cardiovascular illness	141
	– bone demineralization (osteoporosis)	141 & 142
	– arthritis and joint disease	142
	– mental function	142 & 143
	– advice on training	143 & 144
	– weight control	145
Chapter 11:	**Nutrition for the family**	
	– the parents	149
	– the mother and baby; breastfeeding; weaning; the growing child;	150-156
	– hazards associated with breastfeeding	156 & 157
	Hygiene – A diversion	158
	– Semmelweiss; Lister; Public Health; personal hygiene	159-161
	– the growing child	162 & 163
	– school meals	162
	– the teenager	163
	– the young man and the young woman	164
	– the older man and the older woman	165
	– the vegetarian	166 & 167
Chapter 12:	**Functional Food**	171-173
Chapter 13:	**Obesity and overweight Food & Relationship to ill-health**	175-179
	– obesity, overweight, Body Mass Index & liposuction a warning	178-179
	– cardiovascular, gastrointestinal and auto immune disorders	180-182
Chapter 14:	**Other Illnesses associated with wrong feeding**	183
	– obesity, Type II Diabetes, cancer, depression and other mental disorders	185-187
	– example of restoration of health with correct nutrition: case report	224
Chapter 15:	**Food allergy** – Intestinal impermeability testing	189-193
Chapter 16:	**Cancer – some thoughts**	195-199
Chapter 17:	**Examples of different foods**	201-205
Chapter 18:	**The blood type groups** – features in common	207-211
Chapter 19:	**Guidelines –** Cooking techniques and quantities	213-223
Chapter 20:	**Postscript**	225
	Bibliography	229-234

Prefaces

First Preface

As a physician, a clinician, not a nutritional scientist, I cannot claim originality in what I have written in this book. Such knowledge of nutrition as I have acquired and which I would like to share with you, is the result of the efforts of countless dedicated workers around the world; to them goes the credit and my thanks.

My thanks are also due to my many patients, of the past several decades; those very important individuals, who have taught me so much about the practical application of good nutrition.

Many of these, to my knowledge, have helped themselves to have healthier, longer, more active and happier lives by applying the simple principles that we shall be considering together.

Second Preface

People who know me and who had read the first preface, so castigated me for being too diffident that, without altering the original, I am impelled to add a rider.

Having practised medicine for over fifty years, slow learner that I am, I admit to having enhanced my knowledge and expertise and offer to share both with you.

Nevertheless, the words attributed to St. Augustine (AD 354-430) spring to mind:

"It is better to remain silent and be thought a fool than to open one's mouth and remove all doubt."

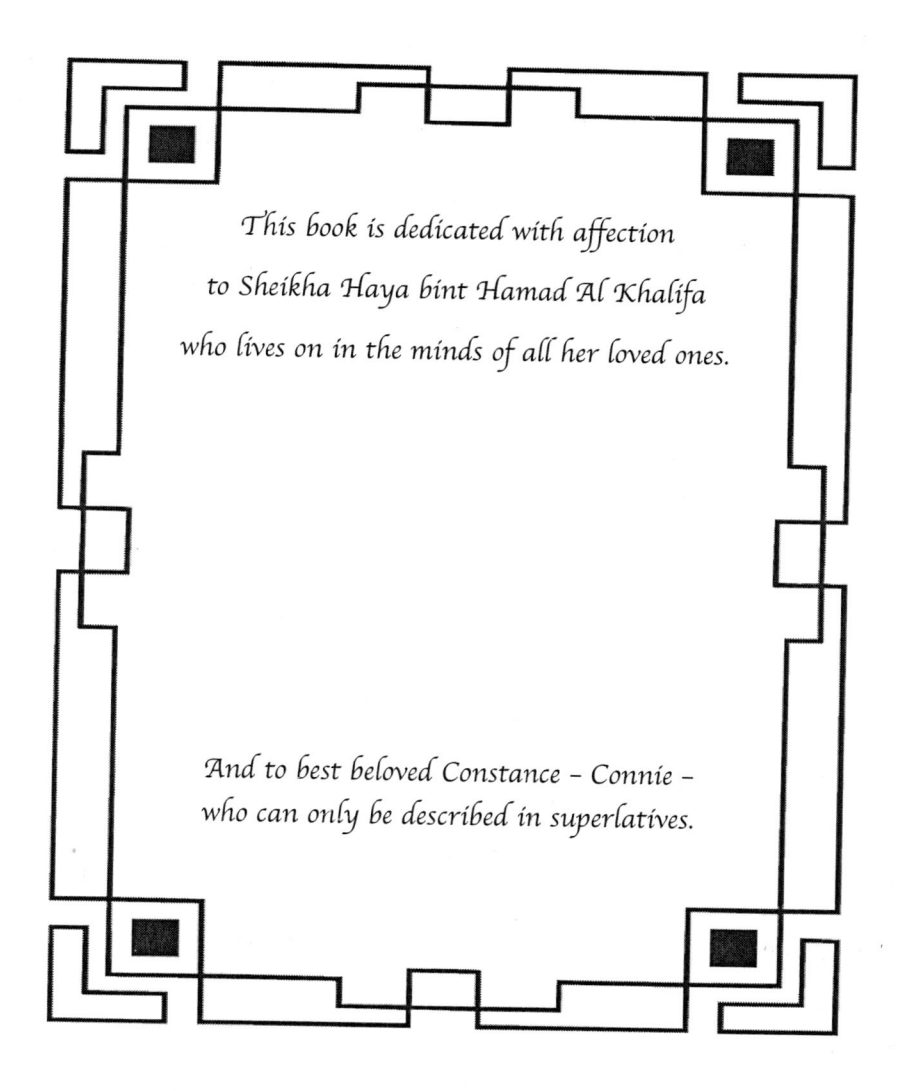

*This book is dedicated with affection
to Sheikha Haya bint Hamad Al Khalifa
who lives on in the minds of all her loved ones.*

*And to best beloved Constance – Connie –
who can only be described in superlatives.*

*There is but one God –
but there are two commandments:
1 Love the Lord thy God with all your heart
and all your soul and with all your mind.
2 Love your neighbour as yourself.*

Food – The Associations

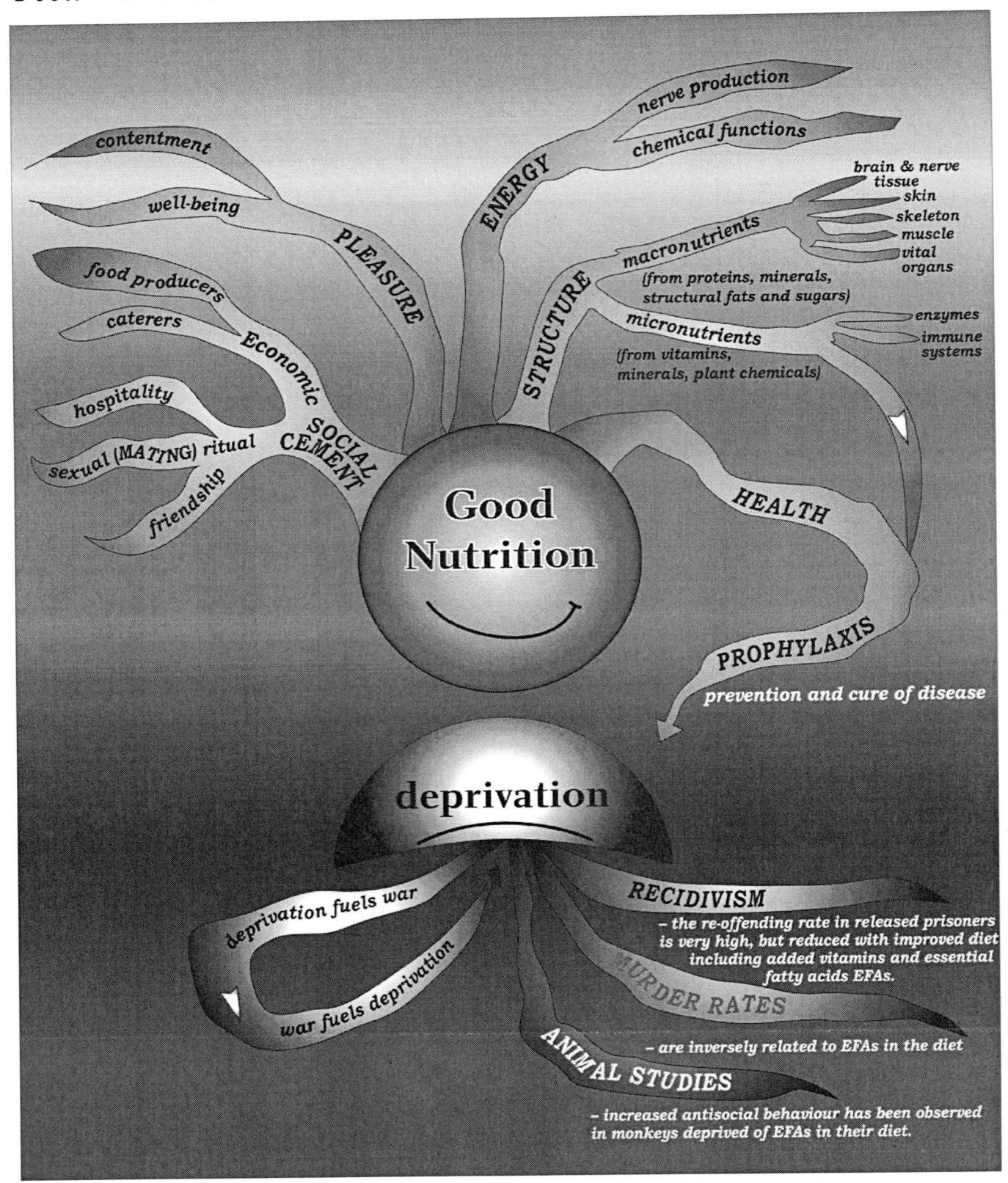

Good Nutrition

- **ENERGY**
  - nerve production
  - chemical functions
- **STRUCTURE**
  - macronutrients (from proteins, minerals, structural fats and sugars)
    - brain & nerve tissue
    - skin
    - skeleton
    - muscle
    - vital organs
  - micronutrients (from vitamins, minerals, plant chemicals)
    - enzymes
    - immune systems
- **HEALTH**
- **PROPHYLAXIS** — prevention and cure of disease
- **PLEASURE**
  - contentment
  - well-being
- **Economic**
  - food producers
  - caterers
- **SOCIAL CEMENT**
  - hospitality
  - sexual (MATING) ritual
  - friendship

deprivation

- deprivation fuels war / war fuels deprivation
- **RECIDIVISM** – the re-offending rate in released prisoners is very high, but reduced with improved diet including added vitamins and essential fatty acids EFAs.
- **MURDER RATES** – are inversely related to EFAs in the diet
- **ANIMAL STUDIES** – increased antisocial behaviour has been observed in monkeys deprived of EFAs in their diet.

Introduction

When starting to write this book, I had first to ask myself "For whom am I writing? Health and nutrition professionals? Interested lay people? parents? Health freaks . . . . . ?"

I decided that it must be for anyone who is involved with food. Whether you are a producer, an advisor, a preparer or you just eat it; young or old, this book is written for you.

Some of what I wish to tell you is personal opinion based on first hand experience of many years in medicine as a practising physician and in agriculture as a practical farmer. Very much more is based on fact; the result of research by acknowledged authorities in many different disciplines, several of whom it has been my privilege to have known personally. These good people have taught me a great deal which I am happy to pass on to you.

Food is a complex subject and some of the discussion in this book deals with some moderately complex science, which I have tried to keep to a bare minimum. Some of this may seem to be complicated to the layman and over-simplistic to the scientist. To the one, I say skip the bits with which you don't want to bother (you may wish to creep back later) and to the other, have patience.

Any single piece of a jig-saw puzzle will give you no idea of the whole design. Only when every piece is put in place will the true picture emerge. Similarly, you may wonder about the relevance of some sections in this book; for instance, how do free radicals or prebiotics relate to the food you eat? Don't worry! Go first to those parts in which you have an immediate interest. Almost certainly each will lead you to another area. Soon all these details will merge, losing their individual identities to reveal the whole picture of what we should understand as food.

Despite everything, the *practice* of good nutrition is very, very simple. You and I know that food is a necessity for us all. It is not simply a fuel, but a supplier of spare parts: materials the body needs for growth and to maintain itself. It should also be fun, interesting and enjoyable.

Fine: why not leave it at that? After all, we do not need a degree in physics to operate a television set or a modern telephone. If we are to take an intelligent interest in nutrition, we need to know a little more. Some food is mostly beneficial and some is not.

How do animals in their normal environment select the foods most suited to their constitution; choosing the right ones and avoiding the wrong, eating what they need and no more? The food they enjoy must be the food they need and, of course, must be available. The same must have been true for our pre-agricultural ancestors, otherwise the human species would have become extinct.

Today, the requirements are no different; availability, attractiveness and, to cover our needs, variety. Yet modern man differs by eating the wrong foods, even shunning the right ones and is prone to overeat. Why?

The answer is that nowadays foodstuffs are produced that satisfy the criteria of availability, attractiveness and variety. They can be coloured,

Introduction
continued

textured, perfumed and flavoured in many ways to appeal, despite being made from ingredients lacking in nutritional value, but providing an excess of calories. They also tend to be addictive.

Another problem (with which our ancestors did not have to contend) is the extraordinary amount of conflicting advice to which people are exposed, whether from professionals, commercial sources, self-interested "gurus" or just plain cranks. No wonder people are not only confused, but often frightened and at a loss to know what to do for the best.

Here are some examples:
- "If you have bread and milk, you have the basis for nutrition." **Not true.**
- "Dairy products (milk etc.) are necessary for calcium and to avoid osteoporosis." **Wrong.**
- "Sugar is necessary for energy, especially in children." **Dangerously wrong.**
- "Red meat is bad for you." **False.**
- "Human beings are intended to be complete vegetarians." **No evidence; anatomical or physiological.**

I intend to put the record straight. In this book I will tell you about the components that, collectively, form what we know as food. From that you will understand the rationale of choosing the diet of our pre-agricultural ancestors. By avoiding what you and I discover to be the wrong foods, the more likely are we to choose and enjoy the right foods and to restore our instinctive ability so to do.

Then you will realise that just as you do not need a degree in physics to work the television, so, **you do not have to be a nutritional scientist to feed yourself correctly.**

For many years, there has been increasing awareness, among doctors and the general public, of increasing unfitness in the population; most particularly in so-called 'developed' countries. Heart and circulatory disease, diabetes, gastrointestinal diseases, cancers of different types and obesity have all been increasing.

The medical profession and pharmaceutical industries have risen to the challenge with the introduction, it must be admitted, of very valuable aids; but, at a price. They may ease the suffering, but rarely cure; often produce undesirable, even dangerous side effects; are becoming increasingly expensive; but, worst of all, causing us all, doctors and patients, to be conditioned to believe that the answer to all our problems lies in a pill; that we are absolved from the responsibility to make any effort on our own behalf.

Many others think differently. For many years, evidence has been accruing that many metabolic diseases, (i.e. not the result of infection or accident), stem from faulty nutrition.

Nothing affects our health and the way we feel more than the food we eat.

A good proportion of our time is spent in the acquisition, preparation and consumption of food; or just thinking about it. The ever-increasing

Introduction
continued

How potty can we get?

One of the maddest recent proposals was contained in an article published in the British Medical Journal; the creation of a so-called "Polypill" to prevent cardiovascular disease and to be prescribed to anyone over 55 years of age, regardless of his or her's being at risk, or not, of stroke or heart attack, (a gift on a plate to the pharmaceutical industry!).

It would consist of six drugs: one, a statin, to lower cholesterol; three to reduce blood pressure; folic acid to reduce homocysteine (considered to be a risk factor for heart disease); and aspirin to reduce the risk of clot formation.

Besides ignoring the reaction of any person to one or more of these drugs and the (sometimes dangerous) side effects, no one knows what other adverse reactions could result from the interactions between the individual components of such a combination.

Such foolish thinking avoids identifying the cause and, therefore, prevention of such illness. It also induces hypochondriasis in people, together with the idea that survival must depend on pill-taking regardless of whatever bad habits we may have acquired.

number of cookery books, diets of every kind, articles in daily newspapers, radio programmes – even tame television chefs – all attest to an intense interest in food. Yet, we are becoming an 'How to do it' society. Technology is taking over. More than 85% of all food eaten today in the U.K. is processed. In some far away factory, ready-to-eat 'complete' dishes are prepared and frozen, ready for the consumer to reheat. Today, fewer people prepare, or are even capable of preparing meals in their own homes, using fresh ingredients.

While a good diet must be aimed at the promotion of health, it must also become a way of life; a source of enjoyment, but not an obsession or religion.

I wish you, dear Reader, Bon Appetit and Good Health!

"If the physician is able to treat with nutrients, not medication, then he has succeeded.

If, however, he must use medication, then it should be simple remedies and not compound ones."

Abu Bakr Mohammed ibn Zakariyya Al Razi, Persian born physician in Baghdad during the 9th century AD and author of *Kitab Al Hawi fi Al Tibb*; a comprehensive book of medicine comprising 23 volumes.

Chapter 1

Origin and Evolution

Origin/Evolution

As far as we can tell, life first appeared on Earth more than three and a half thousand million years ago. Seas at that time would probably have been less than one third as salty than they are today, although it is likely that the first life-forms would have appeared in the shallower waters or estuaries. These waters, too, would have been rich in chemicals, fed from newly formed rivers.

One of the first, and for us, very important known life-form was a bacterium, *cyanobacterium*: a minute single cell organism, able to use the intense solar ultraviolet radiation (which could penetrate the shallow estuarine waters) converting the energy for synthesis – from simple substances, the building of more complex forms and growth. By their biological activity, producing oxygen as a waste product, they gradually transformed the primitive atmosphere, originally devoid of oxygen, into one where animal life could evolve.

Cyanobacteria, sometimes called blue-green algae (although not, in fact algae), predate plants and, initially, were responsible for all oxygen production. Currently they form a large family and, even today, are responsible for producing nearly two thirds of all atmospheric oxygen. One, the tiniest known photosynthetic organism, *Prochlovococcus marinus*, lives in the oceans and – believe it or not – was only discovered as late as 1988.

Pre-human hominids[1] probably date back to at least seven and a half million years, when divergence from the apes occurred. The human genus, however, appeared only a mere two million years ago.

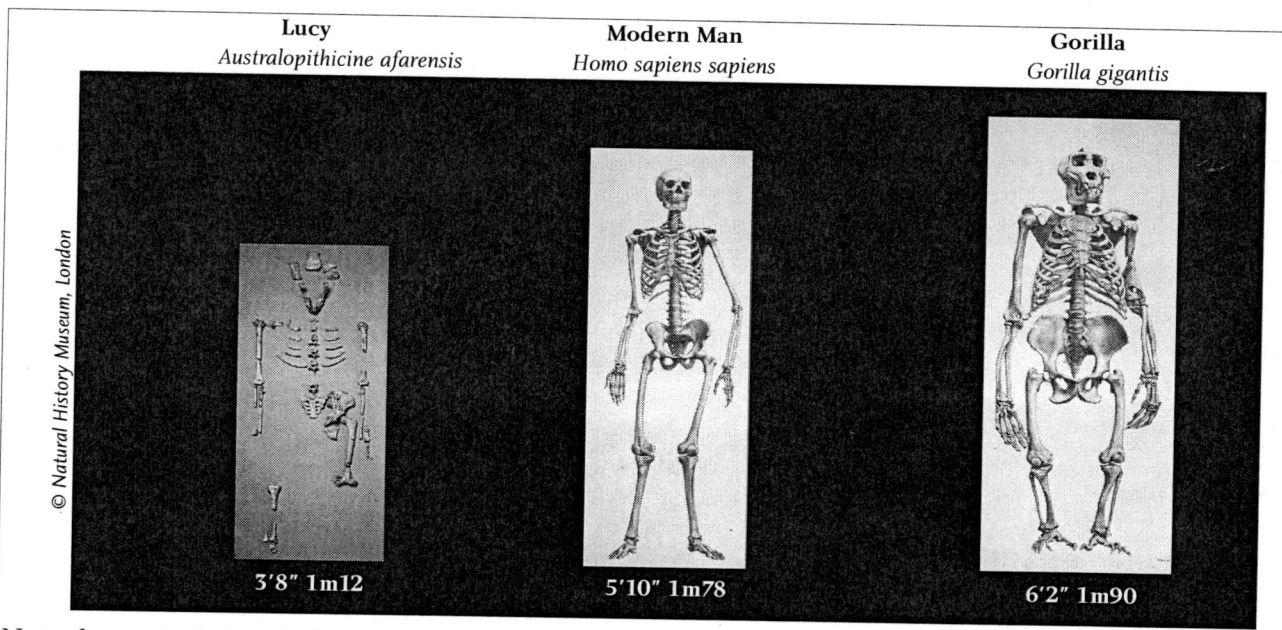

Lucy	Modern Man	Gorilla
Australopithicine afarensis	*Homo sapiens sapiens*	*Gorilla gigantis*
3'8" 1m12	5'10" 1m78	6'2" 1m90

© Natural History Museum, London

Note the conical shape of the rib cages of Lucy and the gorilla, together with the wide bowl-shaped pelvis to accommodate a large digestive tract. In contrast, the thorax of modern man is more barrel-shaped and the pelvis is much narrower although the aperture is relatively much larger and wider to permit the passage at birth of the big head of the human baby.

[1] *an animal of the family Hominidae comprising man and modern apes and his close, now extinct, bipedal ancestors.*

Origin/Evolution

Judging from body shape, (i.e. a rib cage wider at the base than at the top, enclosing a large gut, also from tooth shape and markings), the early hominids were essentially plant eaters. By the time that the first homo (the human genus) appeared, the ribcage had acquired the more modern barrel shape; indicating a shorter digestive tract.

All parts of the mammalian body are made of protein in various forms. The herbivore carries, in one of its stomachs, a veritable factory populated by bacteria. These bacteria, by fermenting vegetable matter, can manufacture proteins. They also produce, from the simple fatty acids in plants, more complex ones; the structural lipids required by all tissues.

Carnivores and omnivores, including cats, dogs, rats and humans, cannot do this. By consuming meat from herbivores, much of the material is, so to speak, "ready-made": a more elaborate and concentrated form of nourishment and so allowing for a shorter digestive tract.

From the time of the early hominids, four and a half million years ago, man's height and weight have doubled, *but his brain size has more than trebled.*

Why the sudden enlargement of the brain relative to body size?

Evidence is that, during the past two million years, man has been a seacoast or lakeside dweller, with characteristics aquatic rather than terrestrial.

- He is the only primate that is hairless; a feature of aquatic mammals. Subcutaneous fat is another shared feature.

- Human babies also, unusually, have subcutaneous fat of a type that aids buoyancy: babies are capable of being born under water[1] and are capable of floating and swimming from birth. [Don't you think that it is peculiar that we should be born able to swim, but have to learn how to walk?] Also present at birth is the "dive reflex", characteristic of diving mammals. When a baby's face is splashed with cold water, the facial (trigeminal) nerve is stimulated, with immediate slowing of the heart rate (bradycardia). This reflex is lost later if not used.

- Humans have a profusion of sweat glands, helping to maintain body temperature when out of water. Additionally, unlike savannah dwellers, we have relatively poor mechanism for concentrating urine; in fact, are very profligate of water.

- We, like most diving mammals and unlike all other land mammals, have voluntary control of our breathing, allowing a swimmer to gulp large quantities of air through the mouth.

- Brain size has increased steadily during the past two million years, with a sudden spurt in the past two hundred thousand years.

(By the way, did you know that only humans and pilot whales have the menopause? I wonder why?)

---

[1] *Michel Odent is a French gynaecologist and obstetrician, who has pioneered a birthing technique, using the natural squatting position, with great benefit to the mother and to the emerging infant. He has also taught a method, now increasingly popular, of birthing under water, where the mother lies in a warm water pool and the baby emerges from under water and (while still attached by the umbilical cord), swims to the surface.*

Origin/Evolution

Nutrition is the Key:

Savannah dwellers develop large bodies in relation to their brain size.

A dolphin's brain at just over 1¼% comes much closer to the human brain.

The human brain is 2% of body weight i.e. 3lbs for a body weight of 150lbs – (a percentage we share with some small mammals such as the squirrel!).

A body is constructed mainly of minerals, proteins and lipids (fats). The brain also requires minerals and proteins, but the bulk of the brain – over 60% – is made from structural lipids. These lipids are made from essential fatty acids, which we cannot make. They, like all other materials, proteins, minerals and other essentials, have to be derived from food.

The two essential fatty acids needed are linoleic (omega 6) and alpha linolenic (omega 3). Omega 6 fatty acids are common on land, whereas omega 3 fatty acids are most abundant in the marine environment; although some can also be found in certain seeds and nuts (hence the squirrel's higher brain/body ratio).

To put it simply: omega 6 essential fatty acids are important for the development of the cardio vascular system (heart and blood circulation) and, hence, the skeletal and muscular development. The omega 3 essential fatty acids are particularly involved in the development and growth of the brain and nervous system.

Provided with these two essential fatty acids, linoleic and alpha-linolenic, the body can convert them to more complex forms.

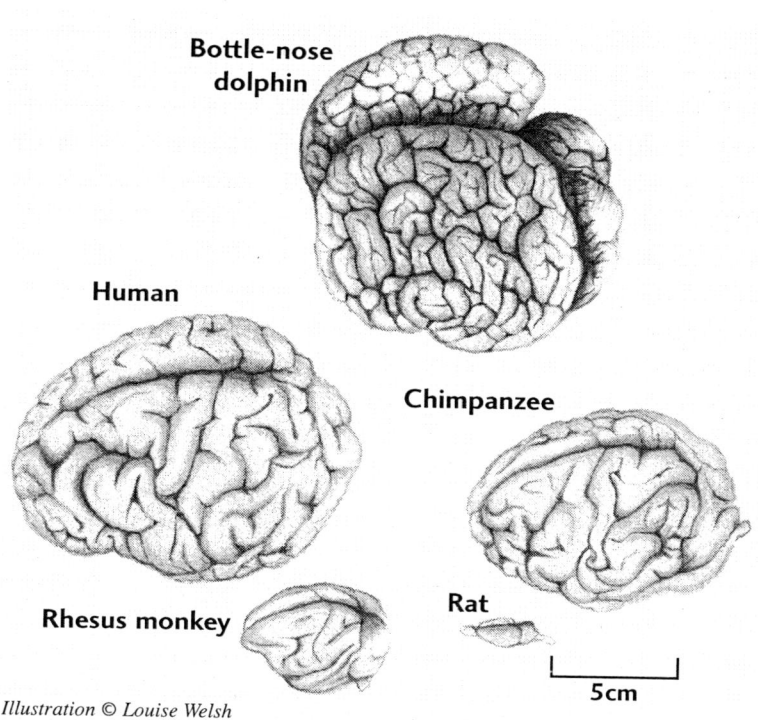

Illustration © Louise Welsh

Bottle-nose dolphin
Human
Chimpanzee
Rhesus monkey
Rat
5cm

e.g.	Rhino	<0.03%
	i.e. 10-11 oz brain in an animal weighing 2000lbs	
	Chimp	0.4%
	Gorilla	0.25%
	Cow	<0.1%
	i.e. <1lb brain in an animal weighing 1000 lbs	

Origin/Evolution
Two pioneers to whom we owe a great deal

The late Professor Hugh Sinclair, M.D., D.M., D.Sc., F.R.C.P. *Director, International Institute of Human Nutrition, Fellow of Magdalen College, Oxford, formerly Director of the Laboratory of Human Nutrition, University of Oxford.*

He was responsible for much innovative work in the field of nutrition, including the role of the essential fatty acids and of lipids in general. Some of this knowledge derived from his observation of the Inuit people among whom he lived for a time and with whose diets he experimented on his own person.

Professor Michael Crawford, Ph.D, C. Biol., F.R.C.Path., *presently Director, Institute of Brain Chemistry and Human Nutrition, London Metropolitan University, Chairman, McCarrison Society, for the study of Nutrition and Health.*

Professor Crawford is recognised as a world authority on lipids and nutrition. Widely travelled, he has argued convincingly on the importance of the essential fatty acids, particularly for the omega 3 group derived from marine sources, in the development of the human brain. Maps showing the human migratory routes (see section on blood group types *page 47*), mostly coastal, support his contention that coastal and lacustrine (lakeside) dwellers would have had greater access to these essential fatty acids, from fish and marine plants than would dwellers inland, where there is relative scarcity.

Chapter 2

Agriculture is not Natural

Agriculture is not natural

Agriculture is not natural

Provocative? Not really. Both my wife and I (especially she) were, for many years, practical "hands-on" farmers. The idea that present-day farming methods are wrong developed with observation and experience; an opinion which is becoming more wide-spread.

Our farm was situated on Exmoor, an upland area in the South-West of England and a natural habitat of the red deer; a most beautiful, if wild, countryside with an annual rainfall in excess of 60 inches (150cm) and a climate that varied from heavenly to savage.

The land covered 650 acres (270 hectares) and ranged in altitude from 1,000 to 1,400 feet (300-400 metres), had its own springs and a small stream where salmon used to spawn and was devoted entirely to grass for the rearing and development of sheep and beef cattle. We also kept chickens, ducks, pigs and horses, including several Arabians.

During our time, we were responsible for many innovations and became known locally as the nearby Government Experimental Farm's "experimental farm"; particularly when our ideas were officially adopted and publicised.

Agriculture is not natural

What is "natural"? Look at wild animals in their own environments and what they choose to eat. We see that they are very selective and can only thrive and breed if their special requirements are met.

The panda, for example, is so specialised that, for food, it can survive on only one particular kind of bamboo. (One wonders if it has not run into an evolutionary cul-de-sac.) There are many animals with very special needs, who would not only refuse to eat any but their proper foods, but would die without them.

Just as we observe the animal in the wild in its natural habitat to learn on which foods it lives and thrives, so we should look at man in his natural habitat to discover his natural foods.

Here we hit a snag. Some of the less specialised species can eat almost anything. Referred to as omnivores, these include rats, pigs and to some extent, humans. Because of their ability to eat (and digest) most foods, animal or vegetable, a problem arises: what are the right foods and are any of the foods that the omnivore can eat harmful? You can see why, when one has the correct information, it is easier to feed those creatures with very specific dietary requirements than it is to identify and select foods that suit a particular species of omnivore.

Man's natural foods: yours and mine

Thanks to the work of archaeologists and paleo-anthropologists, we know that in four million years of evolution man developed into an omnivore eating meat and an abundant variety of plant material: leaves, fruits, nuts, berries. In the last two million years and with the arrival of *homo-sapiens*, seafood assumed greater importance, resulting in the extraordinary expansion of the human brain.

Agriculture is not natural

For the evidence of what is "natural", we must look to those few people left on this earth – so-called hunter-gatherers – who exist, as did our ancestors, on foods not deliberately sown or harvested: some Inuit (Eskimo) away from trading posts; some of the remaining bushmen of the Kalahari desert in Africa and a few Australian aboriginals not yet affected by civilisation.

Their diet is rich in protein and essential fatty acids, moderate in other fats and low in starch. Complex carbohydrates would come from leafy vegetables with very small amounts of sugars from fruits and berries. Included are all necessary vitamins, minerals and other essentials to ensure health and survival of the species.

The Inuit is an exception. During the short summer season there would be a limited amount of vegetable matter. At other times, when a caribou was killed, the stomach would be opened and the vegetable content consumed, together with the meat.

Take note. These are the "natural" foods of at least four million years of human evolution: that means yours and mine.

The products of modern Agriculture do not conform to those eaten by our ancestors: worse than this is the fact that many of the foodstuffs made from these products are linked to many current illnesses; heart disease, obesity, diabetes and cancers, not seen in indigenous societies.

Agriculture originated about twelve thousand years ago in Mesopotamia: latter-day Iraq. It spread gradually, but also seemed to arise spontaneously in other regions (see map). When mankind began to cultivate, the foods produced were cereals and roots because they yielded high volumes of food and

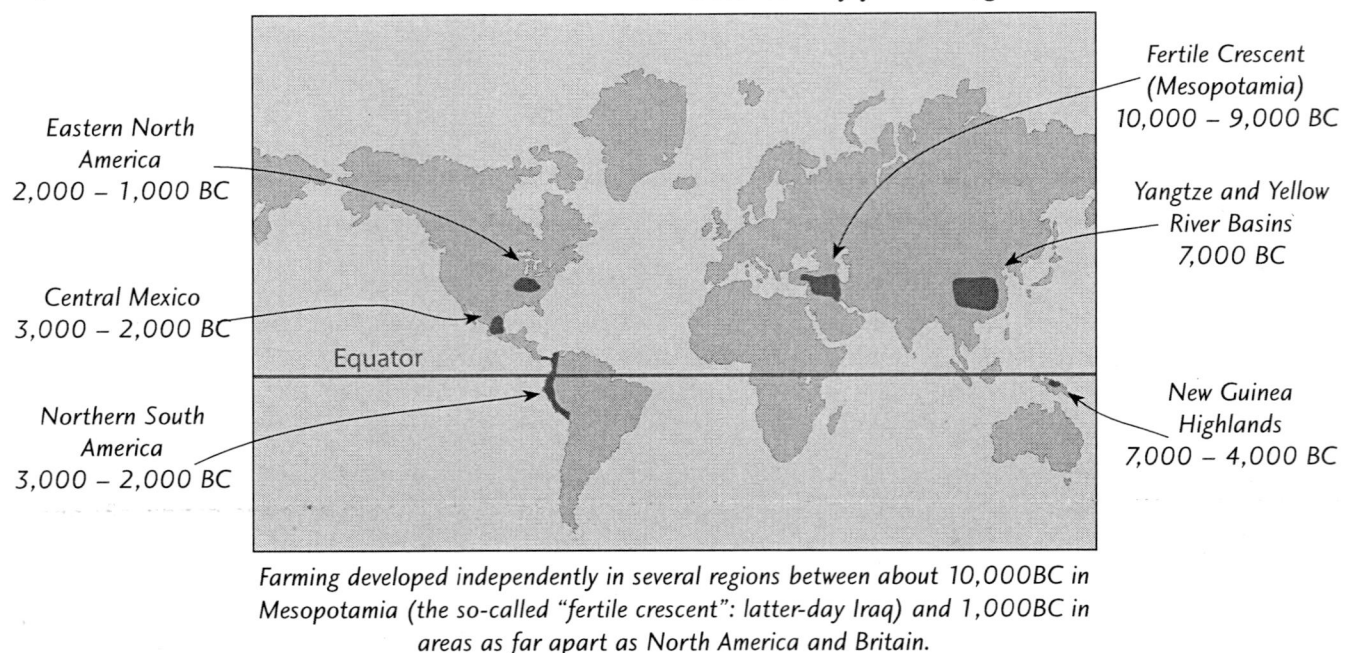

Eastern North America
2,000 – 1,000 BC

Central Mexico
3,000 – 2,000 BC

Northern South America
3,000 – 2,000 BC

Fertile Crescent (Mesopotamia)
10,000 – 9,000 BC

Yangtze and Yellow River Basins
7,000 BC

New Guinea Highlands
7,000 – 4,000 BC

Farming developed independently in several regions between about 10,000BC in Mesopotamia (the so-called "fertile crescent": latter-day Iraq) and 1,000BC in areas as far apart as North America and Britain.

Agriculture is not natural

could be grown relatively easily. They did not then and do not now provide a 'balanced diet'. Cereals and roots still constitute the bulk of agricultural crops grown world-wide today. High in starch, relatively low in protein and fats, especially the essential fatty acids, they bear little resemblance to our ancestral diet. Worse than this: sugar is now the world's largest single food crop; more than double any other including wheat, corn (maize), or rice.

Richer countries have extended agriculture to include animal husbandry for the production of meat and milk.

So, let us take a quick stroll around the farm:

To see cows grazing in a field seems natural enough. But the cow is not naturally a grass eater. It evolved as a forest animal; a browser not a grazer. Have you noticed how level the undersides of trees are in a park where cattle are present? To add insult to injury, the current fashion in the UK is to grow one type of grass, rye grass, for bulk and rapid growth, instead of the mixture of grasses, with different nutritional content and other "weeds" which flourished in old permanent pastures. The grass, too, is harvested for hay or silage before coming to seed, the part in which the valuable essential fatty acids are concentrated. Hence, compared with its wild cousin, the meat in farmed beef is lower in protein and essential fatty acids and higher in saturated fat.

Pigs fare no better. The pig too is a forest animal, a grazer, that digs for roots and eats grubs, insects and fruits such as acorns and beech nuts. In such conditions it is a lean, clean, muscular, active animal. On the farm, pigs are commonly kept confined; often in crowded conditions and fed a high starch diet. As a consequence, it becomes "fat as a pig", with flesh that in no way resembles that of its wild cousin, or that of one of a similar breed, that has been allowed space to roam free.

My wife and I had firsthand experience of this. Although primarily engaged in rearing sheep and beef cattle, we also kept free-ranging Wessex Saddleback pigs who, among other things, were expert in keeping away marauding foxes, especially at lambing times. The pigs were lean, healthy and active, producing successive, large litters of piglets even on the harsh upland conditions of Exmoor, with no artificial shelter.

Chickens, another forest animal, are descended from a type of pheasant: the Jungle Fowl of South East Asia. In its own habitat, a chicken will eat grubs, insects, plant leaves, grasses and seeds. The flesh is lean, high in protein and the fat is largely unsaturated – oily at body temperature. The farmed chicken is kept in crowded conditions, often with space per bird approximating to the size of a page of this book. The conditions are dusty, ammoniacal from bird droppings and unhealthy. The flesh is pallid and flaccid, and the fat, because of the feed, tends to be more saturated.

Eggs, a good food if produced by healthy birds, are nearly all being produced from specially bred birds who are only fit for egg production. The birds are confined to houses in crowded conditions and are fed artificial rations which often contain colourants to improve the otherwise pallid colour of

Agriculture is not natural

The Soil

the egg yolk. After a very short life, being unsuitable to be offered for sale in the shops, the birds are disposed of, presumably to manufacturers of chicken pies, patés and pet foods. The latest information, 2001, is that in the UK, with a population of 60 million, there are 300 egg producers, all with flocks of 20,000 or more, producing 80% of all eggs sold. The remaining 20% is the work of more than 23,000 egg producers most of whom have a flock of less than 100 birds. What is interesting is that the suppliers of birds in the egg-laying industry obtain their chicks from eggs laid by birds living in free range conditions. There are two main reasons for this: firstly, the greater vitality and health of offspring produced and reared in true free-range conditions; secondly, there are, of course, no male birds in an all-female egg-laying house.

Sheep, because of their still semi-wild nature, do not lend themselves to intensive rearing methods and are perhaps less harmed, except where the grasses they eat are in the form of modern monoculture leys[1] rather than the older mixed grass/weed permanent pastures. We also learned from bitter experience on Exmoor that sheep kept in fields of new-sown one-grass-type leys made every effort possible to break out and seek other food. When put into fields of mixed grasses, herbs and deep rooted weeds, they stayed contented even when the field had been nibbled almost to bare earth.

Nevertheless, we all need to continue to grow our food and farmers are needed more than ever. We all, that includes you and me as well as farmers, animal breeders, food producers in general, need to have a complete rethink as to how matters can be made better for all of us.

The Soil

Soil varies in its content of minerals from one part to another: sometimes a deficiency of a vital, beneficial substance, sometimes an excess of toxic substances[2].

Modern intensive farming methods use heavy machinery which cause subsoil compaction and artificial fertilisers which alter the soil structure. The use of heavy machinery and artificial fertilisers also alters the aeration of the soil, reducing absorption of rainwater and increasing surface runoff, which in turn causes erosion. Added to this, the subsurface life suffers. Earthworms, which can tunnel down about 5 feet (1.5 metres) into the subsoil, improve drainage. Unfortunately their numbers can decrease drastically if the soil is managed badly; earthworm numbers can vary from 0.5 million per acre (0.4 ha) on unmanured land, 2.75 million per acre when farmyard manure is spread on the land, to 8.6 million per acre on grassland[3].

You and I really should erect a monument in praise and thanks to these wonderful creatures. We would be dead without them!

---

[1] meadow, pasture or grass; arable.

[2] In some parts of the world, Asia and parts of the US an excess of arsenic in water from wells has caused illness and death in whole communities. In some parts of Britain, iodine is absent in the soil. In the past this caused swelling of the thyroid gland (goitre), hardly seen today since iodine has been added to domestic salt. In other parts, copper deficiency in so-called "teart pastures" is associated with a neurological disorder in sheep called "sway back", nowadays preventable by dressing the pasture with a preparation of copper.

[3] Rothampstead Experimental Station, England

Agriculture is not natural
The Soil

The weight of worms together with various other subsoil creatures and bacteria on healthy land is approximately six times the weight of the animal life supported on the surface. *So for every ton of cattle, sheep or goats that live on an acre of well cared for pasture there are six tons of worms, bacteria and subsoil creatures living under the surface.*

Today, we do have the knowledge of what constitutes "good soil" for the production of good food. There has been and still is much argument

---

Since 1940, five separate assays have been carried out in the UK of the mineral contents of various foods. With the exception of marine foods, which show no change, the reports show that there has been a successive and progressive drop in the mineral content of all land-derived foods; meat, vegetables, fruits, milk and dairy products, grains and, markedly so in manufactured foods. This can only be due to increasing depletion of minerals in the soil.

Current farming practice is to use NPK (nitrogen, phosphorus and potassium) fertilisers to encourage plant growth, with the occasional addition of magnesium and sometimes copper. No attention is paid to the other trace minerals, some of which may not be needed by the plants but are most certainly necessary to the animals (including us) that feed on them. Imagine a supermarket stocked with hundreds of different items. Suppose that as each item was sold out it was replaced only with a can of beans and a toilet roll. Eventually there would be only beans and toilet rolls available. Ridiculous? . . . . perhaps, but that is what is being done to our land. Apart from the depletion, there is a build-up of phosphorus and the excess nitrogen is polluting water courses and rivers.

The spreading of tanked slurry, mostly associated with dairy herds is another factor. Such slurry is potentially dangerous, carrying a heavy load of disease-producing bacteria as well as other contaminants such as detergents, disinfectants as well as antibiotics in the cows' urine. There is also evidence that intestinal worms can survive in tanked slurry. Poisoning the soil in this fashion considerably reduces the subsoil life and so adversely affects the fertility.

Traditional "farm-yard manure" was produced by the in-wintering of cattle in stables on beds of leaves, bracken or straw. The only moisture was provided by the animals' urine. The effect was to harbour bacteria which caused a heating of the bedding (similar to the composting of waste vegetable matter) and so killing off disease-causing bacteria and parasites. The manure when later spread on the ground was, firstly, safer – being less of a health hazard – secondly, returning much of the (now-enriched) original plant matter and mineral content to the soil and thirdly, providing fodder to the vitally important subsoil inhabitants; earthworms, soil bacteria and fungi, among many others.

Agriculture is not natural

The Crops and Trees

about the quality of vegetables and livestock raised by traditional methods using farmyard manures as opposed to artificial fertiliser. For example, there is the careful work of Professor Hartmut Vogtmann, first on the mineral content of vegetables grown by different methods and secondly, the feeding of animals on these differently grown plants, noting the effect on their health, longevity and well-being of their offspring.

> Agriculturalist, agronomist, ecologist, Professor Hartmut Vogtmann is a leader in these fields.
>
> Originally Professor of biological husbandry, Oberwil, Switzerland and then at the Department of Agriculture, University of Kassel, Witzenhausen, Germany in 1994 he was appointed President of the Federal Agency for Nature Conservation in Bonn.
>
> His influence is such that his former faculty at the university has turned 100% to organic farming and is now named "Faculty for Biological Agriculture Sciences". Several new, young professors are all involved in organic farming – even offering an MSc in Organic Agriculture taught in English!

In order to ensure that food grown is of the highest nutritional quality, it is essential to improve communications between researchers worldwide and to pool their knowledge. This information could be applied, making use of local knowledge of climate, access to water and local facilities.

The Crops

Vegetables: Our ancestral diet included a tremendous variety of plants[1], implying that we need a similar variety of chemicals (phyto-nutrients) – not just the vitamins and minerals with which we are familiar – but many others too that have not yet been recognised or their need even suspected. The modern diet, restricted as it is to a comparatively small number of domesticated plants which are grown more for yield, appearance and palatability than real nutritional content, fails to give us the variety of dietary components we need; especially when we remember that the bulk of the modern diet is composed of grains, (totally lacking in the ancestral diet) and roots that are high in starch and low in proteins and essential fatty acids.

[At one time in our lives, we had a walled kitchen garden – oh, bliss! – in which we grew every conceivable vegetable and fruit possible in our English climate – even to melons out of doors on a heap of steaming compost. The worker who helped us to achieve this veritable cornucopia preferred his peas out of a can!]

Part of the answer would be in the development of horticulture with the emphasis on the production of a much wider range of leafy vegetables to suit the locality. A system of rotation would be necessary, involving animals, poultry, sheep, cattle to provide necessary manure and so maintain fertility of the soil.

Yet, despite all our current knowledge, matters have not improved.

---

[1] It has been estimated that of the thousands of edible plants, our ancestors had access to and utilised over 170 different kinds at any one time. Even today, some of the Amerindians inhabiting the Amazon area have been seen to eat over 80 different kinds, in addition to any fish or meat they may catch.

Agriculture is not natural
The Crops and Trees

In 1940, there appeared in Britain a special report: "The Chemical Composition of Foods"[1] published by the Medical Research Council. It describes the mineral and organic content of various British foods; different vegetables, fruits, meats, marine foods, dairy products and some manufactured foodstuffs. This report was updated in 1946 and again in 1960. Two subsequent editions, retitled "The Composition of Foods" appeared in 1978 and 1991, published by the Ministry of Agriculture Fisheries and Food, together with the Royal Society of Chemistry.

Although the list of contents has varied and is not wholly comprehensive, (some not appearing in the early editions), the reports show that apart from marine foods, which show no change, *all land derived foods, vegetables, fruits, meats, milk and dairy products and (especially) manufactured foodstuffs have shown a substantial, progressive decline in mineral content.*

What are the Remedies?

Here are some suggestions:

- review the present use of artificial fertilisers, their effect on subsoil life and the composition, including mineral content, of plants;
- ploughing as a *regular* means of soil cultivation should be abandoned and other less damaging methods adopted; e.g. light discing, direct seeding, chisel ploughing;
- where possible, adopt a modified form of combined farming involving the rotation of vegetation and livestock;
- ensure the return of properly treated (composted, not raw) vegetable and animal waste;
- where practical, use calcified or other dried seaweeds as fertilisers and soil improvers;
- stone dust (free of toxic heavy metals) from quarry waste acts as a slow-release source of minerals;
- intelligent intercropping of plants can reduce, even eliminate the use of herbicides and insecticides;
- a cheap but comprehensive means of soil testing should be readily available to farmers;
- finally, but not least, inclusion of trees in agriculture.

Trees

Of the world's surface, approximately only one tenth is used for food production. Much has been desertified: some by massive climatic change, some by wildfires but much by man's attempts at food production and the coincidental destruction of forest. It has been estimated that, with the aid of trees, *three quarters of the earth could supply our needs*, not only food but of clothing, fuel, shelter and many other basic products[2].

In 1929, J Russell Smith, Professor Emeritus of Columbia University, published his epoch-making work *Tree Crops – A Permanent Agriculture*. His thesis, based on observations in many different countries, states that certain crop-yielding trees can provide useful substitutes for cereals in animal husbandry, as well as conserving the environment. Trees can form part of a permanent agriculture, living as they

---

[1] Authors: R.A. McCance, E.M. Widdowson

[2] *"Forest Farming"* Douglas and Hart. Watkins, London (For other references refer to the Bibliography at the back of this book).

Agriculture is not natural
Trees

do for many decades if not centuries. Being deep-rooted they can bring water and minerals to the surface. Unlike grain crops, trees can be planted on hills and mountains preferably on contour lines where they are not only productive but prevent soil erosion. The labour required is less, being confined to the original planting, grafting where indicated and harvesting the crop. Apart from the many different fruit bearing trees, there are bean and nut producers of many different kinds suitable for human as well as animal food and appropriate for almost every climate. With correct planting, trees can also provide proper conditions for rearing many different animal species. Other trees provide oils, some edible and some for chemical and industrial use, pharmaceuticals (e.g. salicylic acid – the basis for aspirin – from willow bark) as well as providing timber.

In the cloud forest above Santa Cruz in Mexico, an experiment has been carried out successfully for some years in which shade-tolerant coffee bushes have been planted in the forest floor. The result has been to produce coffee (usually a sun-lover, requiring open land) to the benefit of the local community, while preserving the biologically rich cloud forest, its ecosystem and climate.

Mention has already been made of deficiencies of minerals, vitamins and other vital substances in foods today. Allowing that there are areas in which certain minerals are deficient in the soil and that defective methods of food production can cause shortfalls, there is another factor that, until recently, has been almost completely overlooked: carbon dioxide pollution.

Atmospheric carbon dioxide (CO_2) has increased from pre-industrial times, 150 years ago, by 30% and is expected to double by the end of this century. This is wonderful for plants, which by photosynthesis, can use CO_2 to manufacture sugars, starches and other carbon based molecules, while enjoying accelerated growth. In fact, with the doubling of CO_2 it is estimated that crop sizes would increase by 40%, so helping the world's starving population.

Not true!

Studies have shown that with the higher levels of CO_2 plants take up less nitrogen, the key element in the formation of amino acids and, hence, protein. Production of essential fatty acids is reduced while starch production goes up. Uptake of minerals is reduced; zinc, magnesium, calcium, iron, phosphorous, sulphur, selenium, iodine, chromium, manganese, potassium, copper and cobalt amongst others. Plants, collectively, take up some 32 minerals (of which we need at least 26). Individual plants, however, need fewer minerals than we do and relative shortages do not seem to affect plants' ability to grow.

What all this means is that although the *quantity* of vegetable matter – on which ultimately we are all dependent – may be greater, the *quality* will be greatly reduced. **In effect we shall be growing junk food.** The result will be to increase, not relieve, malnutrition world wide.

Much of the answer must depend on a world wide reduction of man-made CO_2. An increased, intelligent use of trees, with their ability to absorb CO_2 together with their other potential benefits, would make a significant contribution.

Agriculture is not natural
Livestock, Fishing and Variety

Additionally, trees have an important effect on local weather and possibly global climate.

Finally, remember that trees in particular are the major converters of solar energy. You and I are being reminded continually that the Earth's non-renewable resources, coal, oil and gas, are diminishing rapidly. **There is yet time, but not much, for all nations to make a concentrated effort to avoid the creation of a world-wide wilderness.**

Livestock:

Like human beings, animals reared in crowded conditions become prone to disease: viral, bacterial and parasitical. Research on deer and other animals also provides evidence of stress. When they are confined in initially adequate space and left in peace with sufficient food, they breed, flourish and multiply. When, however, the density of the population exceeds a certain level, they begin to die.

Post mortem examination has revealed no infection, no lack of nutrition and no other abnormality other than enlarged adrenal glands; indicating that the animal was overstressed.

Intensive rearing and breeding for unnatural growth rates should be abandoned. Apart from the cruelty aspect, the infection rate is high and animals become carriers of dangerous organisms such as Salmonella, chlamydia, lethal strains of E.coli and the quality of the meat is inferior.

Fishing

Current methods of fishing are very wasteful and destructive and need urgently to be improved; with better means of selection of types of fish to be caught and the sparing of others.

At present, many unwanted fish are caught and thrown back (dead) into the sea. This causes depletion of existing fish stocks, not only from overfishing, but by pollution (poisoning) of the seas.

In addition, many sea beds are being destroyed by inappropriate use of newer trawling equipment: all contributing to an impending world-wide shortage of what, at one time, was thought to be an inexhaustible contribution to our human needs.

What we need is variety

Variety is important in foods of vegetable origin and equally so in relation to foods of animal origin: not just beef, lamb, chicken and pork, but also wild or game meats such as venison, hare, rabbit, partridge, pheasant and many others.

Remember also that we should not be confining ourselves to muscle meat; we should eat the offals – liver, heart, kidney, sweetbreads, thyroid and pancreas glands, tripes (and, one day from disease free animals, brains) – which contain many vital substances deficient or absent in muscle meat.

Agriculture is not natural
Apologia

Apologia
Agriculture is not natural.

If one day you noticed that cracks were appearing in the walls of your house, what would you do? Would you call in a builder immediately, or paper and paint over the cracks, or think "this house has stood for so many years, leave well alone" . . . .?

I remember seeing a 200 hundred years old, well-built house in London that must have been shaken by war-time bombing although apparently undamaged and which, some years later quietly collapsed into the street; fortunately without injury to anyone. Nobody had taken note of the developing cracks. (Of all people, the occupiers were building surveyors!)

There is a tendency in all of us (government especially) to procrastinate, to "put things off": not acknowledging any deterioration and, therefore, the need to act until a crisis has arisen – when sometimes it is too late.

The giant super tanker under weigh cannot make a sudden, large alteration of course – even in an emergency; its momentum will take it for several miles before such a manoeuvre can be completed. Similarly, the juggernaut of the present farming industry, on whom we all in some way depend, cannot be made to change direction overnight. Yet, re-routed it must be, but to the *advantage*, not detriment, of all the hard-working people – farmers, agronomists, chemists, manufacturers and others – dedicated to providing food for us all.

The ideas about which I have written in this chapter concerning ourselves and agriculture are based on fact. I have given reasons why change is necessary and will elaborate on them throughout the book.

Such changes as I have advocated cannot be left to government alone. Everyone of us is involved, together with the responsibility for action. Only when individuals act in concert, do the politicians take note. Our organic growers have begun to take the first step.

Our Family, *Homo sapiens sapiens* is unique. If we are to improve our lot and that of future generations, we should act now. Over the next several decades of constructive effort that it will require, we can be sure not only of our survival, but of restoring and enhancing the beauty of our home planet, Earth.

Chapter 3

Food

So what do you want from food?

Definition: [Food] "a substance, or substances, on which a living creature feeds; which, when digested nourishes the body; that promotes growth and activity."

- Better health, physical and mental?
- Sexual vigour?
- Weight-loss/control?
- Improved strength and stamina?
- Greater intellectual capacity?

All relate to correct nutrition.

Dull? perhaps, until you remember that food is a universal source of pleasure; that it should be enjoyable and interesting as well as beneficial.

Food and our Ancestors

When was the beginning for you and for me? at birth? at conception? No; longer than that. You and I have taken at least four million years to arrive here. That is how long it is estimated that Man has been evolving.

For most of that time he was a nomad, a wanderer, finding his food where he could. We know what he ate because nowadays we have the technology to analyse fossilised faeces. Additionally, archaeologists and palaeo-anthropologists have been able to identity large amounts of animal remains, fruit pits and nuts, in areas where human fossils have been discovered.

We know, therefore, that he ate meat. This would have been wild, or game meat, which is lean. Modern farmed meat is, by comparison, obese. Additionally, game meat has a higher protein content and is richer in the essential fatty acids: important structural fats (lipids). Fish bones and shells have been found in abundance in archaeological material dating from 130,000 to 170,000 years ago. Earlier evidence of seafood consumption is lacking, because of the rising sea levels in interglacial times. Seafood (including maritime plants) is much richer in alpha-linolenic acid, the essential fatty acid, the precursor necessary for brain development. It is also a provider of the ready-formed more complex docosahexaenoic acid DHA and eicosapentaenoic acid EPA, the important structural lipids of which 60% of the human brain is composed. (See section on Fats/Fats chemistry.)

It is no coincidence, then, that whereas the brain size of the terrestrial early hominids did not alter for 3 million years, there was a rapid (in evolutionary terms) doubling of brain size among coastal dwellers over the next million years; with an even more rapid rise in the past 200,000 years.

Diet included an incredible range of vegetable matter, leaf, stalk, root, fungus, even flowers(!) – estimated at over 170 varieties. Compare that with our modern diet of a few frozen peas, carrots, cabbage and potato! Even today, in South America, some of the Amazonian Indian tribes have been seen to eat over 80 different kinds of vegetable, in addition to any meat or fish, not to mention insects and grubs, that they can capture.

Eggs would not have been abundant at this time because the wild bird does not lay all year round.

Food

The same inference can be made for fruit, which would have been local and seasonal.

This then is the total diet on which you and I have evolved: a wide variety of meats (not only muscle meat, but offals including liver, kidney, lungs, heart, brains, tripes); a wide variety of fish, including shellfish; and this extraordinary range – not necessarily huge quantities, but variety – of vegetables; together with occasional eggs and fruit – and that's it.

It would be interesting to know how many people existed on Earth one million years ago. Three thousand . . . ten – who knows? Certainly, there was space and an abundance of food (doubtless, with intermittent shortages) both animal and vegetable in great variety.

Inevitably, there followed an increase in population and a diminution – perhaps local absence – in food supplies. Consequently, people began to migrate and, where food continued to be relatively abundant, to form communities. This probably began to take place between fifty thousand to one hundred thousand years ago.

Change

From the nomadic life to agriculture.

With the continuing rise in numbers and resultant lessening of food supplies, Man learned to plant seed and so produce food. He also learned ways of herding, later domesticating, animals for food.

We have been farming, on average, for only five thousand years (probably twelve thousand in Mesopotamia, which includes latter-day Iraq, and only three to four thousand in what is now called the British Isles). It is from this time that the diet has changed: but you and I have not changed. Chemically, we are virtually identical to people born at least twenty five thousand years ago[1].

Decline

From the time that we have been farming, there has been a dramatic reduction of variety of foods previously enjoyed; particularly vegetables, with their contribution of complex carbohydrates, vitamins and minerals. Protein intake declined, both in quantity and variety. Worst of all was the introduction of items into the food-chain for which evolution had not prepared us: sugar, milk and grains[2]. None of these had previously existed in the diet. The widespread use of grains has resulted in a marked increase of starch intake, but diminished protein, vitamin and mineral provision and most importantly, a serious shortage of the essential fatty acids: structural lipids required for the development and maintenance of a healthy nervous and vascular system.

Significantly, stature diminished at this time. Man, one hundred thousand years ago was on average 15cm (6 inches) taller, with massive bones, compared to Bronze Age man farming three thousand years ago.

In Britain, the stature of people continued to decline. Suits of mediaeval armour exhibited in the Tower of London, would not fit a modern twelve year old. The exceptions were among the wealthy

---

[1] See notes on Adaptation pages 46-52

[2] The genus Graminae; the grass family, which includes wheat, barley, oats, rye, rice, millet and maize.

Food

classes who had access to a higher protein intake, mainly meat (King Henry VIII was considered to be a giant). The "traditional" roast beef of England is emotional humbug. Less than one hundred years ago, meat was almost unknown to the general population; the occasional rabbit would provide a treat – but not much earlier than the time of the Roman invasion, when it was first introduced into Britain.

Indeed, as late as the beginning of the Second World War, meat-starved country people in the West of England used to gather snails for food. Named by the locals 'wall fish', these would be roasted on shovels held over a fire and eaten.

Until the middle of the nineteenth century, life expectancy in England of 27 years had been unchanged for two thousand years, since before Roman times. The improvement began with the Industrial Revolution. Having the world's largest navy and mercantile fleet, England began to export manufactured goods all over the world and to import foods from these different countries. At last, there was an increased variety of foods available and a greater supply of protein. At the same time, application of hygiene, with cleaner water supplies and piped sewage, helped to improve the health of the nation. Average height began to rise and life expectancy to increase.

Today, people are becoming even taller. Dentition is remarkably improved, thanks to better dental hygiene and appropriate use of fluoride[1]. Yet, there is, despite advances in medical knowledge, an increase in so-called degenerative or metabolic diseases (not caused by accident or infection) and there has not been any marked rise in life expectancy. Heart and circulatory disorders, diabetes, asthma and other allergies, auto-immune diseases including certain forms of arthritis, obesity and cancers have all increased; not because of better recognition and diagnosis. Doctors have always been well trained in this respect. Cancers, in particular, are on the increase as people do live longer than a century ago, with more chance of their developing; but that does not explain the greater incidence in young people and in children.

So, what is going wrong?

Before answering that question, let us ask another:

How healthy was primitive man and how long-lived?

We can assume that people were, on the whole, well nourished. Food, for the small numbers, was abundant. Vegetation was lush and diverse alongside a highly varied animal population. Additionally, within the last one million years Man was a lacustrine (lakeside) or seacoast dweller having, additionally, access to sea-foods; both fish and plants.

People of one hundred thousand years ago, as revealed by their fossil remains, were taller than those who had later become agriculturalists. Their bones, too, were more massive, indicating that they were more heavily muscled than their successors.

---

[1] See section on minerals: fluoride (fluorine) on page 130

Food
a Sidebar

Here is a puzzle that has, for many years, fascinated many doctors and anthropologists.

While the average height of people in Britain has risen, many of these – particularly the younger ones up to the age of 45 or so – are not built in proportion. Although much taller, they tend to be very slim, light in weight, narrow across shoulders, chest and pelvis, with disproportionately long limbs: notably the legs. The bones are thinner and the joints tend to be lax and hypermobile. The face is narrow with less widely-spaced cheek bones, while the nose is smaller and pinched – often with such restricted airway as to result in mouth-breathing. This facial narrowing leads to constriction of the dental arches, with consequent overcrowding of the teeth and the almost universal need for extraction of the 3rd molar ("wisdom") teeth.

Despite their greater lineal growth, these youngsters lack "toughness", being very vulnerable to infection, subject to allergies and skin problems and deficient in physical strength and stamina. In many cases, there is increased emotional fragility: nervousness, anxiety and depression. Among the women, there is often greater difficulty to conceive (no doubt, compounded by reduced male fertility) and to give birth : the last often the result of a contracted pelvis, necessitating surgical intervention (Caesarean delivery).

This is not a phenomenon affecting only people of the developed countries.

The present-day Masai people, of Africa, appear to share some (not all) of the same problems, which stem more from environmental factors than genetic. Semi-nomadic pasturalists herding cattle and goats, the Masai lived originally in the lush highlands of Kenya. They were renowned as a robust people, fierce warriors, of exceptional height and strong build. They existed on a diet of meat, milk mixed with blood from their cattle, vegetable matter and fruits. Early last century, while the country was under British mandate, these people were expelled from their homelands and forced into lower lying, poor, unproductive land in neighbouring Tanganyika (Tanzania): an area of pestilential diseases.

Food
a Sidebar

The result has been a decline in food quality. Although the diet provides adequate protein it is notably deficient in essential fatty acids: especially omega 3. When a Masai woman knows that she is pregnant, she will practically starve herself to ensure an easy birth (i.e. the infant will be small). One consequence of this is a greater number of premature babies, few of which survive. Of those that survive birth, many die between the ages of 3 to 5 months, from what resembles Sudden Infant Death Syndrome (SIDS): certainly caused by a lack of the essential fatty acids in the mother's diet during pregnancy. Despite this, the Masai people of today do not appear to be so afflicted by the dental and other health problems affecting people of Western Societies. (Perhaps the arduous conditions of their environment are weeding-out the weaker individuals by a process of natural selection.)

Our food in modern Britain, while being abundant in quantity, is markedly different from that on which *Homo sapiens sapiens* (to whom you and I belong) has evolved. Not only has there been a considerable drop in the mineral and vitamin content, but also an imbalance of fats: particularly the essential fatty acids. At the same time, there has been a gross increase of "alien" items (i.e. sugar, milk and grains) and nutrient-impoverished processed food-stuffs which were unavailable to our ancestors.

Now read this:

In the early part of the last century, an American researcher, Dr Francis Pottenger, Jnr.[1], was using cats for his laboratory work. The mortality among his animals was unacceptably high and so, for 10 years (1932-1942), he experimented by feeding his cats with differently prepared foods. *The most deficient diets produced,* in successive generations, *changes in his animals similar to those that I have already described in present-day humans.*

It would be wrong of me to suggest that Dr Pottenger's observations on nutrition (as applied to the purely carnivorous cat[1]), can relate directly to human requirements. On the other hand, the significance of deficiencies of either species producing similar defects in both cannot be ignored.

Here is some good news! Research indicates that such decline can be reversed.

When people affected in this fashion, adopt a correct style of eating, they can experience a considerable improvement in health and general well-being. Should they become parents, their children will have fewer defects. If, in turn, this new generation continues on the same lines, their descendants will benefit even more: as will their children's children.

[1] *"Pottenger's cats, A Study in Nutrition:"* Francis M Pottenger, Jnr. M.D., (1983)

Food

As to how healthy, we can only surmise by comparing with the few, dwindling populations of hunter-gatherer peoples that remain today. The Inuit (Eskimo) people living in their own environment away from trading posts, live on a diet of over 90% meat or fish, with a minimum amount of vegetable (often derived from the stomach of animals they kill, such as caribou). They have low blood pressure, low cholesterol and no heart problems.

I have spoken to researchers who have studied the Inuit people for many years and who have lived with them for months at a time. They told me that, additionally, they had seen no cases of diabetes or cancer. Individuals who had escaped injury or infection lived, apparently, to a healthy old age of 70+ years in spite of the extreme harshness of the environment.

The bushmen living in the Kalahari desert have a diet of over 40% meat, together with leafy vegetables, wild fruits and also have low blood pressure, low cholesterol and no heart problems.

Man's inhumanity to Man

Following the discovery of diamonds in the Kalahari desert and the resultant political pressures, the bushmen of the Kalahari are being evicted; forced to abandon their land and traditional life-style.

They may soon be a thing of the past.

The few Australian aboriginals, who are as yet untouched by civilisation, tend to be coastal dwellers and derive over 40% of their diet from fish and meat. They, too, have low blood pressure, low cholesterol and no heart problems.

This, of course, contradicts current advice about the danger of eating meat.

Primitive man probably had a relatively short life. Most societies, isolated from present-day civilised people, have no defence against infectious disease. A recent example would be that of the extermination of the Patagonian Indians by disease brought by seamen and missionaries from Europe during the fifteenth and sixteenth centuries. Accidents, in the majority of cases, would prove fatal. Additionally, man the hunter would himself be in danger from animals at least as ferocious as himself.

For many years, scientists, anthropologists, palaeontologists and others in large numbers have worked to discover what Man ate during the four million or so years of human evolution. Thanks to their efforts, we do know a great deal about the kinds of food eaten by our ancestors and how that could influence what you and I could and should eat today.

The very early hominids were most certainly plant and fruit eaters as revealed by tooth size, wear and markings. The shape of the skeleton, with its conical thorax (ribcage) and pelvis wider than a modern human's, is evidence of a large gut necessary to cope with the considerable vegetable intake. Most likely, the diet would have been augmented with insects and grubs.

With the arrival of the first *Homo* some two million years ago, the composition of the diet began to alter as meat was introduced in increasingly large amounts and variety; at first almost certainly scavenged but later, with the development of tools, hunted. This diet, richer in protein and more energy-dense, resulted in increasing body size and an increase in numbers.

From this time on, it became clear that the early humans were consuming increasingly large amounts of meat[1]; large accumulations of animal remains and tools for processing have been found at sites of human habitation. Evidence of plant consumption is harder to find because vegetables do not preserve easily except for fruit, seeds and nuts. Nevertheless, it has been estimated that early man made use of over 170 different kinds of vegetable mostly in the form of leaf, root, tuber[2] and berry, contributing something between one third to two thirds by weight of the daily food intake.

The resulting population explosion and depletion of local food stocks prompted a dispersion of people so that, within one hundred thousand years of his arrival, early *Homo habilis* (the "tool maker") was established in widely separated parts of Africa. Within a similar period his successors, *Homo ergaster* and *Homo erectus* migrated many thousands of miles, mostly along coast lines. Originating in East Africa, they travelled to the south of that continent, but also northwards at an astonishing pace (geologically speaking) into Europe and eastwards across the Middle East and the Indian subcontinent into China.

These largely coastal routes of migration introduced a new factor into the diet: maritime foods. Omega 3 fatty acids, essential structural components of brain and nerve tissue and which are comparatively lacking in terrestrial habitats are generously supplied in fish, shellfish, seaweeds and some seashore plants. It is during this time that the size of the human brain, static for some millions of years, began its spectacular increase together with accompanying evolutionary change.

It was about six hundred thousand years ago that our most likely true ancestor appeared. *Archaic Homo sapiens* (later named *Homo heidelbergensis*) was tall, 180cm (5'11") with thick bones denoting heavy musculature and weighing 80Kg (175lb) or more, but with a brain nearly twice as large as that of his predecessors and approaching that of modern man. Apart from in East Africa, evidence of *Homo heidelbergensis* has been found in northern Europe, including the British Isles.

Coincidentally, between two hundred thousand and four hundred thousand years ago, a global climate change was occurring; drought conditions affecting Africa and an advancing ice-age overtaking countries at higher latitudes, with ice

---

[1] *Some authorities estimate that consumption of protein on a daily basis may have been as high as 400g (as much as the human organism can tolerate on a regular basis) equivalent to 2Kg (4½ lb) meat.*

[2] *tuber: underground stems with buds where plant reserves are stored (as in potato or Jerusalem artichoke, sweet potato etc.*

Food

Adaptation

covering most land down to southern Europe. A new, but unrelated species, large-brained *Homo neanderthalensis*, appeared at this time spreading across the whole of Europe, including Britain and eastwards towards Russia. Meanwhile, in East Africa one hundred and fifty thousand or so years ago, another descendant of *Homo heidelbergensis* appeared; taller, 184cm (6 feet) of slighter build, weighing approximately 70Kg (154lb) but with as large a brain. This was *Homo sapiens sapiens* from whom you and I are descended. The aridity of the climate at that time forced these people to disperse rapidly to other regions offering better chances for survival. This is when another factor came into play to which we, today, owe our existence; not so much a continuing evolution as a more rapid phenomenon – *adaptation* – survival of the fittest.

Like the Neanderthals, emigrés from Africa had rapidly to acclimatise to colder, harsher conditions. The darkly pigmented skins that protected from the excessive ultra violet radiation in tropical sunlight would now block altogether the less intense radiation from the weaker sunlight in northern skies and so preventing formation of vital vitamin D in the skin. Individuals with paler skins would, on the other hand, continue to thrive.

Meanwhile, the ice-age continued to advance southwards and winter temperatures continued to plummet. Evidence indicates that the Neanderthals and the earliest modern humans, living alongside each other, unable to cope with such conditions, retreated south as the ice advanced. At about this time, a new, technologically advanced branch of *Homo sapiens* appeared from Eastern Europe. With the ability to clothe themselves and equipped with tools for hunting and fishing, they were able to adapt to and survive in the prevailing climate. The Neanderthals and the earlier modern humans, lacking these advantages, could not and died out, probably between 28,000 and 30,000 years ago.

Adaptation

Present-day *Homo sapiens sapiens* shows remarkable ability to adapt rapidly to differing environments. For instance, dwellers on the Tibetan Plateau living in an atmosphere with half the amount of oxygen as exists at sea level, have oxygen concentrations in their blood almost equivalent to those in people living at sea level. This accommodation has taken place in about 250 generations (approximately 5,000 years). The present-day Inuit (Eskimo) is another example. He can tolerate and remain fit on intakes of protein and fat on which most other races could not survive healthily. Equally, the Inuit would have difficulty in coping with the amount of vegetable matter which for most of us would be a necessity. Yet, the seemingly different pale-skinned Inuit, the coal-black Negro, the desert-dwelling nomad, the inhabitant of the rain forest, the red-skinned Amerindian, you and I, have all been traced to a common ancestor. In other words, we are all, quite literally, similar under the skin. The current differences that we see on the surface are consequences of adaptation to the environment; not mutation or evolution. Of the many branches of *Homo*, ours is the only one left.

The next step would be to use what information we have to discover what is meant by "good nutrition" for every individual; certainly not on the basis that "one size fits all".

What should the present-day Homo sapiens sapiens (you and I) be eating? and why?

I am propounding "normal eating" not "The Strigner Diet" or any other diet so fancily named – Lord forbid! There are too many of them already. Certainly, I have referred to the ancestral diet which evolved as did the human genus. As described it comprised:

- all meats, including the offals[1], in great variety; mostly of herbivorous animals, but including insects, grubs and snails etc;
- fish of all kinds, including shellfish;
- occasional eggs[2];
- leafy green vegetables in abundance and variety, including maritime plants and seaweeds as well as tubers, roots, fungi and flowers;
- seasonal fruits, berries and nuts.

It lacked, totally, grains of all kinds, milk and milk products and most legumes (peas, beans etc.).

There is no doubt that this pattern of eating suits many people living today; perhaps the majority. Indeed in my experience many of my patients have benefited from adopting it. On the other hand, there are many others who are definitely not happy with this regime. One person may be able to tolerate only small quantities of meat, finding it difficult to digest ("sits heavily in the stomach") while another can tolerate only certain kinds but not others – chicken for example. Some individuals can take a limited variety of fish and there are others who can tolerate only relatively small amounts of vegetable and in limited variety. Whereas in the ancestral diet, milk and grains were totally lacking there are individuals who appear to be able to use these items to their benefit, when for the majority of people, they would be detrimental.

Why should there be these differences? If we all sprang from a common ancestor, our body chemistry should be identical, but it is not. Wherever you are, in the world, look at the people around you. Note how different one is from another, in height and build, colour of skin, facial structure, hirsute or hairless. You would be quite justified in wondering if each belongs to a different species. *Yet every one of us is a member of the one and only survivor; Homo sapiens sapiens*. Like it or not, we are all brothers and sisters.

Adaptation – Survival of the fittest

The differences, not only of appearance but also of body chemistry, are due to *adaptation* (a more rapid process than evolution) over the past 40-50,000 years; the result of migration and the consequent pressures imposed by different climates, flora and fauna. Alongside the changes in chemistry,

---

[1] Offals are valuable sources of important nutrients and comprise: liver; lights or lites (lungs); heart; kidney; sweetbreads (pancreas and thyroid glands and testes); tripes; intestines (chitterlings – English, andouillettes – French). At present, because of the fear of spongiform encephalopathies (BSE for example), not brains.

[2] Eggs would not have been abundant as the wild bird does not lay all-year-round. My experience with patients shows that the number of eggs eaten at a time matters less than how frequently. Some people who eat eggs daily can develop an intolerance, which does not happen when restricted to two or three times in a week.

Food

there appeared a new phenomenon: different, mostly incompatible, blood types. Beginning with the original, universal type O, there developed some 15-25,000 years ago a variant, type A, to be seen along the migratory routes from Africa to the Far East; later into Western and Northern Europe. Then, 10-15,000 years ago, another variant appeared along the routes north and east to the Indian subcontinent, the Himalayas and Russia. This was type B, to be found among the nomadic peoples occupying the vast areas between Europe and Asia, with some penetration into Eastern Europe. The newest and rarest, appearing only 900-1,000 years ago, type AB, seems to be a hybrid; the result of intermarriage of peoples with type A and type B blood.

What has all this to do with the food we eat?

As each blood group developed, there were associated changes in body chemistry, which we see today, imposed by the necessity to combat the pressures of environmental changes. For instance, although there exists no evidence of agriculture 25,000 years ago, the inference from archaeological evidence is that man's very success in hunting was forcing the consequently larger populations to flee areas depleted of food and to move to more lush areas. These larger communities would, over time, reduce the animal population, but with abundant vegetation would be able to survive. This period saw the beginning of domestication of animals for food. Over several thousand years, adaptation (following Charles Darwin's rule of survival of the fittest) produced individuals with a greater capacity to live and to thrive on a more vegetarian diet, but a lesser capacity to cope with most meats and some fish. These, type As, had developed increasing capability to make use of some seeds (grains) and legumes, absent in the earlier type O.

Later still, people of the blood group type B appeared (remember, we are considering changes taking place over a time span of 5-10,000 years), mostly in much harsher conditions. They appear to have acquired even greater adaptability to extremes of climate and to variety in food; coping well with most meats, fish, most vegetable but not legumes. It is probable that these people were the first to domesticate animals for food and so to develop an ability to make use of altered milk (soured milk, cheese, yoghurt), but not grains, seeds and some nuts. Judging from the evidence of where subsequently farming developed independently, (see map) it is likely that they were also the first-time agriculturalists.

The newcomer, type AB, has predictably, some of the advantages as well as the disadvantages of both types A and B, being able to cope with moderate amounts of lean meat, offals and game, most fish excluding crustaceans and some flat fish such as plaice and sole, but like type B, able to use altered milk products. Type AB individuals seem to tolerate nearly all vegetables and fruits (except citrus), most nuts but limited grains.

The differences between each blood group type are not as clear-cut as I have described. There are variations within each group because there have developed several subtypes. Nevertheless, they are sufficient to explain the contrasts one sees in one person's reaction compared with another's; whether to items of food, drugs, chemicals in the

Food
Adaptation and Dogs

environment, or types of exercise. Why, for instance are types O and B more susceptible to influenza compared to types A and AB and yet have a lower overall rate of of incidence of all types of cancer?

Our immune systems are very sophisticated affairs, equipped with numerous defensive substances, antibodies, produced in response to the action of a foreign body, antigen[1], such as the toxin of a parasite. The development of the different blood groups was accompanied by many adjustments to the host's antibodies to cope better with changing chemical challenges in unfamiliar environments. Hence, the blood groups have different antigens and produce specific antibodies to other blood types[2].

These differences also relate to a very wide range of proteins found in foods: the lectins. Many of these lectins would be compatible with your blood type and so be beneficial. Others, incompatible, would render that food harmful, with varying degrees of toxicity and so capable of doing a great deal of damage; to red and white blood cells, intestinal lining, joint surfaces and nerve tissue.

So, although the ancestral diet would be the correct prototype, it is necessary to consider the individual requirements that have been imposed by the development of different blood types. This we can examine together in a separate section on nutritional patterns.

---

[1] Antigen: any substance that stimulates the production of a defensive substance (antibody).

[2] Dr Karl Landsteiner, an Austrian physician, first discovered and described in the early 1900s the interactions between the various blood groups. If you are interested, some references will be found in the bibliography.

An example of adaptation, as opposed to evolution is wonderfully illustrated in another species, familiar to us all: Man's faithful companion, Dog. DNA studies reveal that all dogs, of which there are four distinct genetic groups originating at different times and places, have a common ancestor: the wolf.

Informed guesswork suggests that early humans learned to tame and domesticate wolves, perhaps as long as 120,000 years ago. Almost certainly, they would have begun to choose for particular qualities by selective breeding and crossing, with eventual genetic divergence of the dog from the wolf.

The fact that, at present, there are more than 800 breeds of dog in the world with such enormous differences in shape, size and character as exist between the Yorkshire terrier and the Saluki, the German-Shepherd and the Old English Sheepdog, the Pekingese and the Bulldog for example – one species with the wolf – is entirely the result of human manipulation, which is continuing.

Most of these changes have been achieved during the past 14,000 - 22,000; much too fast to be the result of evolution.

© Natural History Museum, London

Food

The accompanying maps depict some of what we surmise about the emergence and dispersal of the various blood group types throughout the world.

They can only be approximate as they are based partly on archaeological and paleoserological evidence and partly on conjecture. Nevertheless, they can be helpful towards a better understanding of adaptive differences in appearance masking a biological similarity; why, for instance, the blood of a black type O is more likely to be completely compatible with a white type O, but not with a black type A or B and vice versa.

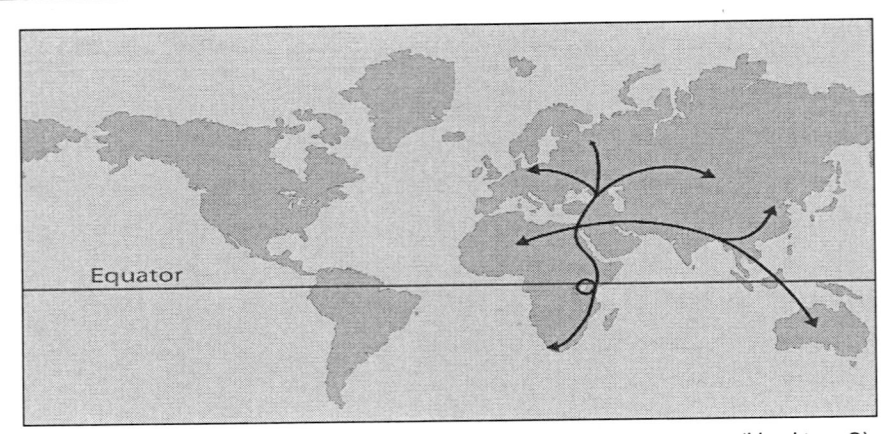

Map 1 showing probable migratory routes of early *Homo erectus* and *Homo sapiens* (blood type O). 400,000 - 25,000 years ago.

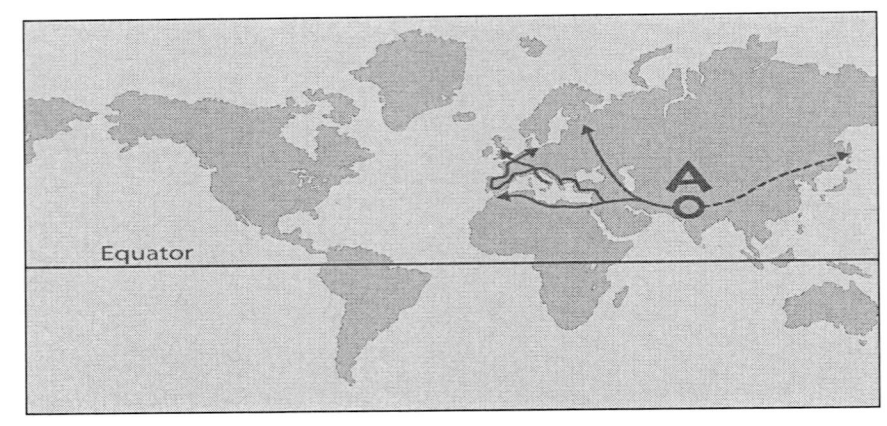

Map 2 showing migratory routes of blood group type A. 25,000 - 15,000 years ago.

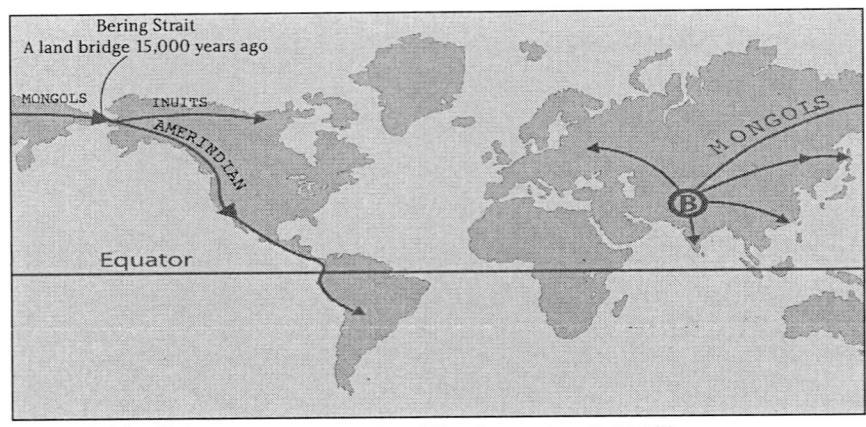

Map 3 showing migratory routes of blood group type B. 15,000 years ago.

Food
Lectins and Tissue Types

Lectins

They are usually proteins which are found in many plants and, therefore, in many foods. Many of these lectins correlate to specific blood types, thus confirming Man's adaptation to different foods during his history of migration.

Lectins, also known as protease inhibitors, are essentially poisons. They are part of the plant's defences against insect attack – even minor damage stimulating generalised production through all parts. They cause stunting of the growth of the predator, thus limiting possible harm. Organically grown vegetables, not protected by insecticide chemicals, would be richer in lectin content than other commercially grown crops.

In the body, lectins can cause cells with incompatible antigens[1] to agglutinate (stick together) causing damage, for example to blood cells, the lining of lungs, digestive tract and blood vessels. These hazards are avoidable by staying with foods suitable to your blood type. The other advantage is that lectins can alert the body's defences and act as part of its armoury against cancer. Malignant cells are many times more easily attacked and destroyed by lectins than are normal cells.

[1] **antigen:** *any substance that stimulates the production of an antibody.*
antibody: *a defensive substance produced in an organism in response to the action of a foreign body such as a bacterium, virus or the toxin of a parasite.*

Tissue types

The differences between the blood groups with regard to food are broadly true. They do not, however, explain the way in which individuals of the same blood group react differently to the same foods (e.g. why some people of group O can tolerate grains and pulses, or some people of group AB tolerate citrus fruits while others do not).

Just as individuals have different blood groups, so they also have different tissue types. There are so many more of these than there are blood groups that it is difficult to be able to match tissue types between two people, even if they share the same blood group (how often have you heard or read of appeals for a compatible donor for a patient – often a child – to make possible a bone-marrow transplant?). Whilst there is only a handful of blood types, there is a myriad of tissue types.

Among the diseases characterised as "auto-immune disorders", such as rheumatoid arthritis, there are correlations between certain tissue types and particular diseases within this group. Similarly, some disorders are seen more frequently in certain blood groups; for example, stomach cancers occur more often in people of blood groups A and AB.

We must, therefore, accept that tissue type is just as important with regard to adaptation to particular components in the diet (and vulnerability towards certain illnesses, if we stray off the path) as is the blood group. Fortunately, in practice, this does not necessarily mean that selection of foods for your particular type is made more complicated. Although there are several sub-types for each blood group, the pattern for each one to be described is much the same. Three sub-types for each group[1], identifiable by laboratory tests, provide clues for individual variations. *The original blood group, O of our early ancestors, sets the pattern for all.*

[1] subtypes:
Rhesus positive and negative.
Secretor and non-secretor
(Lewis a and b) M and N antigens

Food

Adaptation

Adaptation is very much more rapid than previously thought.

Recent research at the Rowett Research Institute near Aberdeen in Scotland, the University of Ghent in Belgium, as well as studies at the University of Toronto in Canada and the University of Arkansas in the USA, have all shown that the chemicals in the food we eat can alter the function of our genes and, therefore, increase or decrease our risk of disease.

The effect seems to stem from an alteration in the balance of the more than one thousand types of bacteria which we carry in our digestive tracts and upon which our well-being depends. Despite the work of many pioneers in this very important field, our knowledge and understanding of this relationship is at present incomplete.

It has, however, been known for a long time that mothers who are themselves unfit and lacking essential nutrients during pregnancy, are likely to produce children with greater risks of disease in later life, such as heart disease, obesity or diabetes. Similarly, their children will in turn inherit these tendencies, but magnified.

The converse is also true. If such a malnourished mother is supplied with sufficient supplementation to compensate for the deficiencies in her diet, she will give birth to children whose risk of developing such diseases in later life is much reduced or even absent. Furthermore, these children's children will derive even greater benefit.

Evidence from many independent researchers indicates that the more adequately nourished are *both* parents *(see chapter on Nutrition for the Family – the parents, page 149)*, the healthier and the more protected from future disease will be the resulting children and, in turn, their descendants.

Although ideally, good nutrition should begin *before* conception *(see again chapter on Nutrition for the Family – the parents, page 149)*, it is comforting to know that even after years of malnutrition and resulting chronic illness, the body can and does respond positively when the nutritional pattern is corrected; an effect I have been happy to see repeatedly in many of my patients.

Should we be eating our food raw or cooked?

It depends entirely on what food we are considering.

Meat and fish, for example, are very easily digested raw as, in the adult, are eggs. In fact, like the carnivores, humans do not even have to chew meat or fish to a fine consistency. The healthy stomach is well equipped and can deal easily with meat or fish swallowed in lumps.

Nearly all fruits and nuts are best eaten raw, but do require more thorough mastication, for which our teeth are well-designed. "Soft" leafy vegetables of the types used in salads[1] can all be eaten raw with benefit, but do require to be chewed

> (lettuce, watercress, endive, rocket, purslane, celery, mushrooms; herbs, such as parsley chervil, mint and even what, today, many people consider to be weeds such as dandelion, fat hen, Good King Henry – even flowers)

thoroughly to break down the cell walls and to release the contained nutrients; a good reason for taking time to enjoy a meal!

---

[1] A very informative, well-written and inspiring book listing over 100 plants is *The Salad Garden* by Joy Larkcom. ISBN 07112 03660

Food
What's going wrong?

Most other vegetables are best cooked.

Although little physical evidence exists of the use of fire by our ancestors prior to three hundred thousand years ago, the implications are that it must have been in use in the time of *Homo erectus*, nearly two million years ago; a period which witnessed the incredible growth spurt of the human brain. *Homo erectus* was more than half again as big as his predecessors but his teeth and digestive tract were smaller; suggesting that the nutritional content and energy value of the food were greater. Cooking vegetables breaks down the (to us) indigestible cell walls, rendering the contents more easily available; in fact, equal to what would otherwise be obtained from twice the amount of the same eaten raw.

Last but not least, cooking offers a means of sterilising foods, so reducing the risk of infection – bacterial, viral or parasitical. Cooking can also destroy toxins present in some plants (e.g. Fava beans, Manioc) so rendering them safe to eat.

A recent study in Germany, of people who ate raw foods[1], revealed that one third suffered from chronic energy deficiency and that half of the women were either amenorrhoeic (without periods) or were suffering from menstrual irregularities. It was calculated that to obtain sufficient energy to maintain even a leisurely life-style, a raw-food-eater would have to consume a weight of food equal to 9% of body weight. In other words, a person weighing 70kg (154lbs) would need to eat 6.3kg (nearly 14lb) weight of vegetables in a day!

So, back to the question - what is going wrong?

In the abundantly fed populations of the world, three signs of illness, previously associated with the few more affluent societies such as Britain and the United States, are emerging: high blood pressure; raised levels of fats, triglycerides, in the blood; and insulin resistance – acquired loss of effectiveness of the vitally important glucose-controlling hormone, insulin.

These are the precursors of coronary heart disease and diabetes. The causes? Faulty diet, fatness, physical inactivity and, to a much lesser extent, genetic inheritance.

Let us consider the culprits:
SUGAR
Sugar, in the diet, is a poison[2]

It has been taught, erroneously, for some time that an excess of saturated fat in the diet is dangerous. What has not been generally acknowledged is that sugar[3] can be worse.

Sugar is something that none of us should be taking in any quantity. It formed no part of man's food in the millions of years of evolution. Yet, consumption of this substance, unknown even as recently as the time of Ancient Greece (when there was no word for it in the language), has rocketed alarmingly.

---

[1] Authors: Richard Wrangham and NancyLou Conklin-Brittain

[2] Poison: "any substance which, when taken into or formed in the body, destroys life or impairs health: any malignant influence." *Chambers Dictionary 1998*

[3] Sugar includes honey, syrup, treacle (molasses)

Food

The Dangers of Sugar

Two hundred years ago, in Britain, the average consumption of sugar was about 2 lbs (less than 1 Kilogram) per person in a year. Today the average is about 2 1/2 lb (approximately 1.2 Kg) *per week!* This is fact.

Not all of the sugar eaten is added to the tea or to the coffee. Much of it is hidden. It is present in soft drinks, heavily advertised, of which more and more are being drunk[1]; as it is in heavily advertised "snack bars" and other sweets. The present-day fashion of trying to subsist by "grazing" frequently on pastries, pizzas and sandwiches is an added factor. Look at the cookery section of any women's magazine and you may find a paragraph or two on the preparation of the main course of a meal, while two or more pages are devoted to the preparation of cakes, biscuits, desserts, jams and other sweets.

Nowadays, most manufactured foods, including preserved meats and vegetables, have sugar added to them.

The danger is that sugar is habit forming. Children exposed in this way to sugar, very quickly acquire a "sweet tooth" with a consequent desire for sweet foods usually starchy in character and deficient in essential nutrients[2]. The result is a decline in health, overweight leading to obesity and development of type II diabetes. Mental illness, behaviour problems, learning defects, depression are all frequent accompaniments of the resulting malnutrition.

Of course, our bodies use sugar, principally glucose, as one of its fuels, but prefer to make it from the food we eat. Taking in sugar (or for that matter any kind of refined carbohydrates – starches – which, during digestion are turned rapidly into sugar) can upset the control mechanism, which is designed to regulate supply.

When we eat our food, a gland, the pancreas, releases the hormone insulin into the bloodstream. This stimulates the tissues, especially the muscles, to take up glucose coming from the digestive tract. This is stored in a more concentrated form, glycogen, by the muscles for their own use as a fuel. The liver can also store a small quantity of glycogen, approximately 100 grams (about 3 1/2 ounces), mainly to be used as a brain fuel. Insulin also prevents the liver from releasing fats, triglycerides used as fuel, while fats from digestion are present.

Excess sugar in the diet, more especially when we "graze", snacking on high energy foods and drinks, promotes prolonged high levels of insulin in the blood. The liver ceases to inhibit triglyceride secretion, leading to insulin resistance in the muscles, interfering with their ability to take up glucose from the blood, so that blood sugar levels rise, eventually leading to the development of "late onset" (type II) diabetes. In addition, the circulating fats become biologically altered, causing them to stick to the linings of the blood vessels, reducing essential blood flow and increasing the risk of developing blood clots.

---

[1] *In the UK, consumption of cola drinks alone, quadrupled in the five years 1998-2003*

[2] *In the UK, especially in the north of England and Scotland, thousands of infants under five have to undergo multiple extractions – often seven or eight – of milk teeth: the result of poor diet and sugary drinks in feeding bottles.*

Food

"Pure, White and Deadly"

The answer: firstly, to limit the number of meals in a day to two, three at most[1]; secondly, to avoid sugar and starches and to derive the complex carbohydrates from leafy vegetables, roots and pulses. From these the body can manufacture the glucose it needs without overwhelming its control systems. Although fruits contain sugars, these are released relatively slowly and the effects seem to be modified by other substances in the fruits.

Fructose, fruit sugar, is present in relatively small amounts and is dealt with differently from glucose; in the proportions present in fruits, it may be beneficial. In larger amounts it is dangerous, being shunted directly to the liver to form fat. Table sugar, sucrose, is digested to 50% glucose and 50% fructose. "Sugar free" or "diet" drinks are frequently sweetened with corn syrup, derived from maize, which is high in fructose. It is also added to breakfast cereals and to a wide variety of processed foods. Incidentally, dates are one fruit with high levels of fructose. They may be of value to people living on a restricted diet, such as the Bedouin in hot desert conditions, but for people in more affluent conditions should be used in moderation.

The current fashion for the frequent drinking of commercially produced fruit juices in large amounts adds to the problem. We are told that 1 litre (approx. 2 pints) of juice is derived from 1.5Kg (approx. 3½lb) of apples, or 15 oranges, or 10 grapefruit. Who in his senses would eat that quantity of fruit in a day as well as the food he needs? Yet many people are quaffing these juices by the litre. Apart from the dangerous amount of sugar (some "pure" fruit juices have had sugar added) – and now significant quantity of fructose – much of the valuable fibre and other phyto-chemicals are absent. Fruits, although valuable sources of some vitamins and minerals are lacking in "body building" materials; proteins and essential fatty acids.

A recent survey conducted in the USA on the effects on children noted that those consuming the largest quantities of juices were below average in physical growth and mental ability. I assume that their lack of development was, in part, due to their being deprived of correct and sufficient sustenance.

Sugar is the chief cause of cardiovascular disease[2] as noted 30 years ago by Professor John Yudkin[3] in his book "Pure, White and Deadly". Atherosclerosis, narrowing of the blood vessels due to fat deposition; coronary thrombosis, due to clot formation in the arteries supplying the heart muscle; venous incompetence.

For years it was considered and still is by many, that high blood levels of cholesterol are causative of heart and circulatory disease. Therefore, it was considered to be important to avoid use of

---

[1] This rule does not apply to the growing child, where energy expenditure is very high in relation to weight and where there is greater need for the materials necessary for growth.
Like a motor car with a small fuel tank, children need 'filling up' more frequently; four or five meals a day in the first 10-12 years would seem to be appropriate.

[2] Rated by The World Health organisation, WHO, as the No. 1 health problem, followed by cancer.

[3] John Yudkin, Professor of Nutrition at London University. A clinician, researcher and world wide lecturer, he had the courage to voice opinions contrary to those widely held at the time.
Experience has shown many of his predictions have proved to be correct, although at the time the relevant laboratory evidence was not available.

Food
Dr Weston Andrew Price

In America, Canadian born dental surgeon, Weston Andrew Price was puzzled to note that dental decay and associated illnesses were almost the norm among his "civilised" patients, yet rarely seen among people of less affluent "primitive" societies.

This remarkable man, having retired relatively early, undertook a series of expeditions between the years 1931 to 1936 that took him, quite literally, all over the world. Together with his wife, he made very close observations of different races ranging from Inuit (Eskimo) in northern Alaska to Gaels in the Scottish Isles. He also visited various groups in Africa as well as making a study of the Amerindian societies in Canada, North and South America; included were studies of the indigenous peoples of many Pacific islands, ending as far south as Australia and New Zealand.

Dr Price was intrigued that despite the differences between the various cultures there was a remarkable resemblance in the perfection of the dental arch, facial structure, teeth and evidence of excellent health – even in harsh environments – which he attributed to their ethnic diet; always riverine, lacustrine or marine. Wherever these different people were introduced to the modern, Western diet, their children suffered marked deterioration, not only in jaw formation, but also smaller sinuses, narrowing of the nose with reduced airway and the consequence of respiratory disease. Some children also exhibited other skeletal abnormalities and all lacked the vital good health of the parents.

Because of the remarkable commonality of these effects in so many different cultures, Dr Price concluded that the origin could only relate to deficiencies in the modern diet and unnatural, excessive sugar consumption. His researches, together with hundreds of fine photographs, are incorporated in his book *Nutrition and Physical Degeneration*. It is a classic; not just about teeth but particularly the role of nutrition and its relationship to health.

(See bibliography page 230 and appendix).

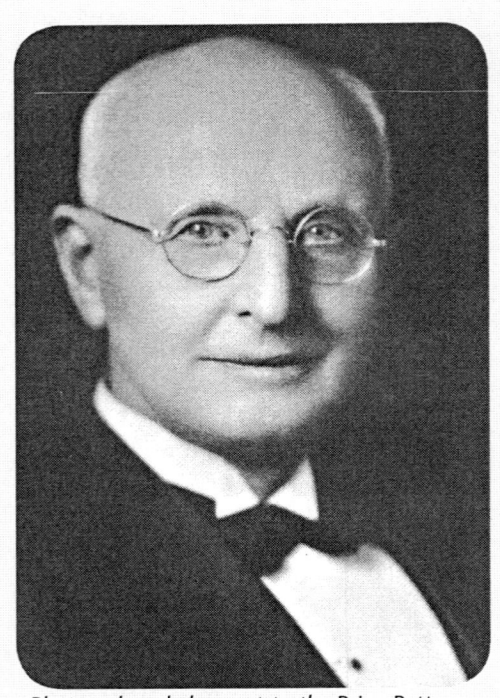

Photo acknowledgement to the Price-Pottenger Nutrition Foundation

Food
Sugar and mental disorders

cholesterol-containing foods, especially eggs, shellfish and, to a lesser extent, meat. In fact use of these foods makes very little difference. The amount and the kind of fat in the diet is more important. Some fats (and as has been mentioned, sugar can be involved in their formation) can raise cholesterol levels significantly. On the other hand, the unsaturated fats (including olive oil, which is mono-unsaturated) and especially those essential fatty acids of the omega 3 group, will reduce levels of cholesterol.

Diabetes, already mentioned, often but not always associated with obesity, is also linked to the body's inability to cope with sugar in the diet.

Over-consumption of sugar correlates to the worrying increase in mental disorders. The B complex group of vitamins are actively involved in the metabolism of glucose; the conversion of glycogen and use as a fuel. With constantly high levels of blood glucose, the vitamins become depleted. As they are all required for proper function of the brain and nervous system, the resulting lack can lead to a variety of nervous disorders; including fatigue, memory loss, lack of concentration, depression and certain forms of schizophrenia[1]

Varicose veins constitute another prevalent disorder. In primitive societies living on their original diet, the incidence of varicose veins is approximately one in two thousand, which accords with genetic inheritance. In the UK, it is ten percent – fifty times as much – and this seems to be entirely related to sugar intake.

What is worse, the incidence increases generation by generation. If the parents, who have inherited the factor, continue to eat sugar, the chances of their children's developing varicose veins are increased. If the children maintain a similar sugar intake, the chances of their children's developing varicose veins are further increased.

It is, however, a process that goes both ways. If parents, who have varicose veins, stop using sugar in their diet the chances of their children's developing varicose veins are reduced, and if they, in turn, don't take sugar in their diet their offspring, also, will have a lower risk of developing varicose veins.

For example, it used to be thought that waiters, or waitresses, on their feet all day were more likely to develop varicose veins. In fact, all round the world, there are communities where much of the work is done standing, yet there is no sign that these people develop varicose veins as a consequence.

Haemorrhoids (i.e. "piles") are also related, but there are additional factors involved, including dietary faults that can lead to constipation.

---

[1] *Much work on the therapeutic value of correct application of minerals and vitamins in mental disorders has been pioneered by Dr Abram Hoffer of Vancouver, Canada and the late Dr Carl Pfeiffer of Princeton, New Jersey, USA, amongst others.*

Food
Milks

Milk

There is no such thing as milk, singular. There are milks, plural: Human milk; cows' milk; cats' milk; elephants' milk. Each one is unique, designed only for the infant of that species.

Recent DNA research indicates milk *tolerance* first appeared in humans in the higher (northern) latitudes about seven thousand years ago; suggesting that milk intolerance is the norm.

As an example, a well-formed human baby at birth may weigh 3.6 - 4 Kg (8 - 9 lb). At six months of age, while being breast-fed by its mother, it will have doubled its birth weight. Having raised beef cattle, I know that a calf at six months on its mother, would have at least quadrupled its birth weight, the reason being that cows' milk contains a large proportion of protein for body building and a large amount of saturated fat, a concentrated fuel, for the energy for growth. Human milk contains much less protein, less saturated fat, but a variety of essential fatty acids designed for building brain and nerve tissue. You see, the baby's brain continues to grow for several years after birth, whereas the cow's brain does not.

Another fact: In Britain, about 50% of people lose the enzyme lactase, for digesting lactose, a sugar peculiar to milk and not found elsewhere. Commonly, this occurs at an early age, between one and three years. Indeed, a proneness in those children who catch frequent colds, earaches, sore throats, chest infections is an almost certain indication of a developing milk intolerance. In countries further south, such as Mexico and China, about 80% of people lose the enzyme, while in some parts of Africa, 100% lose it. I have spoken to some missionaries who discard the milk powder that is sent to them, because it makes the children ill. Curiously, although initially the problem is an inability to deal with milk sugar, subsequently it develops into an inability to deal with milk proteins. This means all milk products; milk in all forms, all kinds of cheese, cream, ice cream, yoghurt and all foods to which any of these may be added.

So when the question, *"where do I get my calcium?"* is asked, ask another: *"Where does the cow (or the cat, or dog, or gorilla, or elephant) get its calcium?"*

The answer is: **"In all the foods you eat, with the greater variety the better".**

Remember, no animal takes milk after it leaves its mother.

Grains

Grains, members of the grass family, pose another kind of problem altogether. Whereas they would have been absent in the palaeolithic diet, grains, since the advent of agriculture, have become increasingly prominent. Today, they are dominant in the diet of nearly all populations, with a proportionate decrease of other nutrients, notably meat, fish and vegetables. Although a reasonable source of omega 6 essential fatty acids, important structural lipids for body building, grains are seriously deficient in the omega 3 group, responsible for the development and maintenance of the brain and nervous system[1].

Another issue: the body's mechanisms for dealing with carbohydrates are designed to cope with the very complex forms that occur in leafy vegetables, roots, tubers and berries. The starches in grains are present in much greater concentrations and being less complex are broken down more easily to basic sugars. These are rapidly absorbed in large amounts, resulting in excessively high blood sugar levels and putting a strain on the apparatus designed to keep the blood sugar levels within correct limits. [2]

Matters are made worse by the currently universal custom of "refining" i.e. discarding most of any protein and vitamin content, leaving behind material that is almost pure starch; solely a source of energy, but devoid of practically all items required for repair and maintenance; including the essential fatty acids. Consider the logic behind the refining of flour, so removing any vitamins and trace minerals and then adding back some – not all – in arbitrary fashion ("fortifying") to make it more "nutritious".

Consider something else. Current evidence indicates that, apart from some adaptive changes already described, our bodies have not changed chemically within the past twenty five thousand years. Yet, in that time, we have introduced into our diet, in increasingly large amounts, these alien[3] substances that had been totally absent in the millions of years of evolution.

---

[1] See chapter on Components of Food – Fat pages 72-79.

[2] See chapter on Components of food – Carbohydrates and the Glycaemic Index pages 80 and 81.

[3] Today, "alien" should include the thousands of additives, vegetable oils and hydrogenated fats that adulterate foods. (Fruit oils such as avocado and olive should be considered to be acceptable).

Chapter 4

Food for thought

Food for Thought

Mens Sana in Corpore Sano:

**Mens Sana in Corpore Sano :
A Healthy Mind in a Healthy Body**

Dirt has often been described simply as matter out of place.

Perhaps we might consider mental illness simply as emotion out of place.

I tend to regard the logical part of ourselves as looking at a picture or photograph in black and white and the emotional part as adding something so that we now see the same picture in full colour.

We need emotions; even those that feel unpleasant.

It is not abnormal to feel anxious or sad, angry or frightened if there is good reason, however uncomfortable we may feel. What is not acceptable is when such emotions arise for little or no reason; where they become excessive and cannot be shaken off, even if the cause is removed; where they interfere with normal function such as sleep, appetite, digestion, blood pressure, breathing and prevent one from thinking clearly and coping with other matters; where they lead to irrational behaviour, possibly endangering one's self or others.

Mental illness has been increasing all around the world: most noticeably, over the past 50 years, in the developed, industrialised nations and, nowadays, apparent in those developing countries that have been introduced to and are adopting the so-called "Western" style of eating.

In the United Kingdom, we are seeing a rapid rise in mental afflictions among young people; conditions include post-partum (after birth) depression, suicide and violence. Suicide in young men of ages 15-34 years has doubled in the past 30 years; the rate being four times higher in men than in women. The most severe of such illnesses – schizophrenia – almost unknown in aboriginal societies, has similarly increased.

When you consider that the developed nations have greater access to food and have more available, sophisticated medical treatment, you might expect the opposite. The truth is that those native cultures that have been studied (today, regrettably, increasingly rare), living by hunting wild game, fishing and vegetables – wild or cultivated – have shown very little evidence of those mental illnesses affecting modern society; schizophrenia occurs at only around 1 case in 1,000 of population, which would accord with the genetic rate. Interestingly, if one of a pair of identical twins (offspring from a single egg) develops schizophrenia, the chances of the other's developing the disease are only 50%: arguing that environmental influences are major factors.

Violence, terror and mental illness go hand-in-hand with incorrect nutrition.

Whatever we choose to call the Soul or the Mind, it has to operate by way of that electro-chemical instrument that we call the Brain.

Food for Thought
Mens Sana in Corpore Sano:

This remarkable creation, superficially a lump of fat and water and averaging just over 3lb (1.4 kg) weight in the adult human male, can produce – quite silently and without fuss – an amazing energy output amounting to 20% of the total output of the whole resting organism!

Controlling all the vital functions, it depends on the rest of the body for all the materials needed for it to work without error. Ultimately, these materials must come from the food that we eat. If the food is in some way inadequate, we can expect brain function to be affected.

For example: When the diet is low in omega 3 essential fatty acids (found largely in fish and other marine foods), illnesses such as post-partum depression, suicidal tendencies, bipolar disorders (schizophrenia, manic depression) are more common. In New Zealand, where the average individual consumption of fish is 40lb (18kg) in a year, depression affects six per cent of the population. In Japan, on the other hand, where the individual average consumption of fish is three times as much, depression affects only one person in a hundred. Of course, other variables of environment and culture must also be taken into account. Nevertheless, the difference is striking.

Other illnesses and phenomena include rises in attention deficit hyperactivity disorder ADHD, autism, dyslexia, dyspraxia, recidivism and murder[1].

The foetus in utero is very sensitive to deficiencies in the mother. The omega 3 essential fatty acids (not only alpha-linolenic, but also the long-chain polyunsaturated eicosapentaenoic and docosahexaenoic acids), omega 6 arachidonic acid together with folic acid and selenium (among others) are crucial for placental and fetal tissues, the formation and construction of cell membranes as well as the formation and development of the brain and nervous system before and after birth[2].

Deprived infants, even if they survive birth and the early growing years, are more likely in adulthood to suffer from heart disease and risk of coronary thrombosis. Other risks are the development of insulin resistance, obesity and type II diabetes.

> [There exists a phenomenon that demonstrates that some emotions are chemical in origin. The advent of depression, for no apparent reason, lasting for weeks or months in someone with no previous history of such, has long been recognised by physicians as a precursor of impending heart attack. If recognised in time, appropriate treatment can avert an attack – with the disappearance of the depression].

Nowadays, the effects of chemicals in foods (whether naturally occurring or artificial) on mental

---

[1] Joseph Hibbeln MD; Bernard Gresch.

[2] A continuing supply of these vital nutrients is essential, not only to ensure the development of a completely well-formed infant "in full working order," but subsequently, a completely healthy adult.

Food for Thought
Mens Sana in Corpore Sano:

function and mood are becoming more widely recognised.

My first awareness occurred while farming in the 1960s. I needed to contact a neighbouring farmer. I knew that I would not find him at his farm, or the market. The only place of which I could be certain was a particularly remote inn on the moor. When I arrived, the place was empty of customers, but the inn-keeper assured me that my neighbour would certainly come.

While waiting and talking, our conversation turned to discussing the arguments and violence that occurred among some of his customers. The inn-keeper was quite definite that the majority of fights occurred among those people who drank beer or whisky. Other people might over-indulge in other kinds of alcoholic drink and behave stupidly, but would rarely become fighting drunk. A similar observation – equally definite – was made to me by a man who managed a truly enormous public house in the east of England.

In other words, it is not the alcohol alone, but other substances present in the drink that can cause the particular mood change. This could also explain the crowd violence that occurs at some social gatherings: football matches for example.

Perhaps we should not be too surprised. The *predictable* effects of some drugs such as hashish, coca, opium, have been known for centuries. We also know that today, we have chemical agents which can calm, excite, induce sleep or wake us up and, in many other ways, alter mood. That items in our food can produce similar effects had not previously been seriously considered.

Many paediatricians are familiar with the child who goes into tantrums – even rage, sometimes lasting for hours – after eating a piece of bread, or an iced "lolly" (water ice) coloured and flavoured artificially. Other vulnerable children show other signs such as hyperactivity, attention deficit, sleep disorders and mood changes such as fearfulness and unhappiness: additionally, physical symptoms include unexplained headaches – including migraine – abdominal pains and bowel disorders. It is unfortunate that these children are often considered to be grossly abnormal and treated symptomatically; frequently with mind altering drugs.

The culprits? Not surprisingly, items in our present diet that did not exist in the ancestral food chain and that can affect the many susceptible individuals among us: milk and milk products; grains – especially wheat – and many of the numerous synthetic colourants, flavourings, perfumes and texturizers used in manufactured products.

The remedy: restore the correct food programme, avoid the culprit foods (and, of course, sugar); as far as possible, use only fresh foods – meat, fish, vegetables and fruits – organically grown;

Food for Thought
Mens Sana in Corpore Sano:

avoid, where you can, manufactured foods. It may be necessary to check for acquired deficiencies and use what supplementation is indicated.

The result: a return to normal behaviour and health. Children usually respond very rapidly.

Notice that the elements that comprise our evolutionary, pre-agricultural nutrition – meat, fish, leafy vegetables and fruits are rarely to blame. The exception is the occasional person with an acquired susceptibility/allergy; perhaps to eggs or a particular type of fish or vegetable.

The lesson: Although we are rarely able totally to control our environment and the burdens that it may impose, it is possible to preserve a healthy mind in a healthy body *(mens sana in corpore sano)* by maintaining a correct nutritional regime, appropriate exercise and adequate sleep.

Chapter 5

Components of Food

Components of food
Protein

Some of the things of which we are made

> What are little boys made of?
> What are little boys made of?
> Frogs and snails
> And puppy dogs' tails,
> That's what little boys are made of.
>
> What are little girls made of?
> What are little girls made of?
> Sugar and spice
> And all that's nice
> That's what little girls are made of.
>
> *Nursery rhyme*

Preface

In this section I have included some basic biochemistry for reference. This is not absolutely necessary for understanding the concept and so, if you wish, may be ignored.

As I mentioned earlier, food is not simply a fuel, but a supplier of spare parts; materials the body needs for growth and to maintain itself.

Imagine that you wish to build the house of your dreams. You have the blueprint for the design (architects' drawings, plans) and a supply of sand, cement, metal ores and other basic raw materials, plus a source of power.

Switch on the power and watch as, first, these basic materials are transformed into more complex ones and then a minuscule version of the house appears and begins to enlarge; fabricating walls of one kind of material, the roof in another, windows and doors of others, electrical wiring, pipes for plumbing, paints, carpets, curtains until the full sized mansion is complete in every detail.

Realise that all the materials needed, including the paints, the pigment for colouring, yarn for all the soft furnishings, carpets and curtains, even the energy required, are being produced by the house itself from the basic raw materials.

Continue to imagine that this dwelling, using these same very basic materials, can renew worn paint, repair broken roof tiles, renew carpets and other fabrics as they wear; in other words, maintain itself in complete good order. A dream? Yet this occurs in each of us, from the time of conception, birth and throughout life. Of course, for this to take place correctly, a proper supply of the right materials is necessary.

They include:

Proteins, fats, carbohydrates, minerals, vitamins, fibre and, not least, water.

In the pages that follow I hope to explain, with a minimum of technicality, the role of each and how, together, they form *food*.

Components of food

Protein

Practically every tissue in the body is made of protein of some kind of which there are thousands. The protein, from which skin is formed is different from that in arm muscle, different again from heart muscle, mucous membrane and so on. For that matter, protein in any tissue is different from the corresponding tissue in any other species.

In the human body, proteins are built from substances called amino acids of which there are twenty. Eight are termed essential (nine in children), because they cannot be synthesised in the body. Originating in plants, formed from nitrogen in the soil, carbon, oxygen and, sometimes sulphur, they are combined into larger molecules to form protein.

Just as the 26 letters of our alphabet can be joined in different sequences of differing lengths to form thousands of different words with different meanings, so too, can the amino acids be joined. Depending on the order of joining and the numbers involved – often several thousands – so are formed different proteins with different properties.

I mentioned earlier that many animals, ruminants and other herbivores, can utilise simple plant proteins to elaborate the more complex ones needed by their own bodies. Plant proteins often lack some essential amino acids and have imbalances in others. These deficiencies can, to a large extent, be made up by increasing the variety of plant material eaten. Animal proteins tend to be more complete and, in that respect, more adequate in the diet of omnivores, including ourselves; necessarily so in the diet of true carnivores, e.g. the cat family.

In the process of digestion, proteins in the food are broken down to the component amino acids. The body can then rearrange them to form its own new proteins as they are needed. Some amino acids are also required to perform separate, individual chemical functions in the body; but this is outside the scope of what we are now considering.

How much protein?

About one fifth of the weight of any lean farmed meat (or fish) is protein. Wild, or game, meat may have slightly more because there is less fat between the muscle fibres. About one quarter is carbohydrate, and the rest is a mixture of fats, minerals and water. The content of fish is similar.

There is, as yet, no consensus as to how much protein we need on a daily basis. Estimates vary between 40 and 100 grams. In the United Kingdom, the level has been set arbitrarily at 70 grams. It seems, on the basis of much research, that the requirement remains the same, whether one is engaged in very heavy physical activity, or is sedentary. An exception would be a woman who is pregnant or is breast feeding a baby; in each case having to meet heavy extra demands on her constitution to provide of materials for growth of the uterus, placenta and herself, as well as the child.

Components of food
Protein

The assertion has been made that too much protein in the diet could damage the kidneys by forcing them to break down the excess. As is generally the case, however, the kidneys, like other organs in the body, have vast reserves and can cope very well with much higher intake of protein. This is evident amongst different populations in the world, who live very healthy lives. For example, Inuit, living in their own conditions, may have over 90% of meat or fish in their diet; the Bushmen of the Kalahari desert over 40% meat; ranch workers in Australia and Argentina have a very similar intake, amounting to 200 grams or more of protein daily. Protein is, of course, a source of nutrients for growth, repair and maintenance. Any excess can, however, be converted to carbohydrate and used as fuel.

It would be reasonable to assume that people who are physically more active would eat more food. As protein rich foods are generally better supplied with minerals and vitamins, they should also contribute to a more complete and healthy diet.

Specific Dynamic Activity

Ingestion of a meal containing protein is followed by a rise in biological activity – the metabolic rate – of the body which is maintained for several hours.

This property, peculiar to protein, has been recognised for decades and termed Specific Dynamic Activity. The intensity of this activity varies with the origin of the particular protein, being lower in vegetable proteins and higher in those derived from meat or fish. The most marked effect results from proteins originating in wild or game meats, including wild birds such as partridge, pheasant, mallard, snipe and animals such as deer, hare, rabbit and, unexpectedly, camel.

The advantages of Specific Dynamic Activity are the enhancement of physical and mental activity and because the effects are long-lasting, an increase in stamina. Hunger is, therefore, kept at bay and because the body is active and at the same time more "fuel efficient" the risk of obesity is low.

Please note that what we are considering here is not great quantity, but the *quality* of protein.

Components of food
Fat

Fats are water insoluble organic substances, solid at room temperature (25°C or less), whereas oils are liquid. Essentially the word "fat" has the same meaning as the word "lipid" and either can refer to the whole group.

Dietary fat is absolutely vital

- It is a major source of energy.
- Just as protein is involved in the composition of all tissues in the body, so, in different forms, is fat; for all cell structure and for the formation and function of cell membranes.
- It is a source of essential fatty acids used in cell structure and the formation of hormones.
- It is a carrier of the fat soluble vitamins and pro vitamins.
- It is involved in the control of blood lipids.
- Without fat, most food would lack palatability and texture.

Although almost as diverse as proteins, fats can be divided in two categories:

Neutral fats including the triglycerides, (stearic acid from beef, for example), cholesterol (of which more later) and the vitamins A, D, E and K.

The triglycerides, the composition of which will vary with the diet, are also known as storage fats. They constitute the most important energy reserves in the body and are also a source of essential nutrients. They form the adipose tissue under the skin and, in excess, become involved in the problem of obesity.

Structural fats, consisting mainly of phospholipids and cholesterol, are extremely important in the formation of all the soft tissues in the body. They comprise over 60% of the structure of the human brain and nerve tissue. Many of the structural lipids have a peculiar property in which part of the molecule is hydrophilic (miscible with water) and part is aliphatic (miscible with fat). They are termed amphiphilic (attracted both ways) and are responsible for the way in which cell membranes function.

The fatty acid component of phospholipids is crucial to their properties and function in biological membranes. The composition of fatty acids in the phosphoglycerides is specific to tissue and species.

Although not as easily affected by the diet as are the triglycerides, gross deviation can produce imbalance in some of the fatty acids.

Subsequent pages are intended to describe some very basic facts relating to the structure of different kinds of fat.

With so much current misinformation and the resulting confusion, it is necessary to have a proper understanding of the importance of fats in the diet and the effects on your health.

Components of food
More about Fats

Because of so much misinformation and misunderstanding, fat is thought of as something "bad" and, therefore, to be avoided. *Nothing can be further from the truth.* Although briefly considered in the section of components of food, perhaps a little more explanation would be useful.

The total weight of various fats (including subcutaneous adipose tissue) in the body of an "average" fit person of 1m75 (5'10") in height and weighing 70kg (154lb) is approximately 10Kg (22lb) in "dry" weight; one seventh of the whole!

It consists mostly of triglycerides, the bulk being stored subcutaneously (attached under the skin) where it acts as an insulator and, like the fuel tank in a motor vehicle, is the main fuel reservoir for the body. Linoleic acid (18:2, $n6$) accounts for 1Kg and alpha-linolenic acid (18:3, $n3$) for about 200g. Made by plants, not by animals or man (although the last comes also in food from animal sources), they are termed "essential" because they can only come from the food we eat.

Our energy is derived from three major nutrients; protein, fat and carbohydrate. Whereas protein can supply 4 Kilocalories[1] per gram (Kcal/g) and carbohydrate between 3.7 to 4.2 Kcal/g, fat has the highest energy value of 9 Kcal/g.

In developed countries (but not exclusively) dietary fat contributes 35 to 45% of energy, with protein providing 10 to 20% and carbohydrate the remainder. In the developing world, however, consumption of fat in the diet may only provide 10 to 20% of energy, with a correspondingly low intake of protein.

Although most dietary fats are triglycerides (made up of fatty acids which may be saturated, mono-unsaturated or polyunsaturated and of varying chain lengths), the types can vary according to origin. For instance, in Asia dietary fat is mostly of vegetable origin, whereas elsewhere animal fats would form half or more of the total intake. In societies where lipid intake is very low, the dietary fats would be predominantly phospholipids; the structural fats found in all cells, animal or vegetable.

It seems, therefore, that we may be able to maintain a good state of health on widely differing intakes of fats, both in amount and type. Let us first consider some of the functions of fat.

Functions of dietary fats

They are:

- major sources of energy;
- indispensable sources of essential fatty acids;
- obligatory for the composition of structural fats, for all cell structure and for the formation and function of all membranes;
- as structural fats, essential to the formation and function of brain and nerve tissue;
- components for the formation and composition of hormones;

---

[1] *calorie: a unit used in expressing the heat or energy-producing value of foods. It represents the amount of heat required to raise the temperature of 1 gram of water (at 15°C) by 1°C.*
A Kilogram calorie (Kcal or Calorie) = 1,000 calories.

Components of food
More about Fats

- conveyors of fat soluble vitamins, e.g. A, D, E, K and pro-vitamin A (the carotenoids);
- controllers of blood lipids, including cholesterol;
- modifiers of appetite through hormone production by adipocytes (fat cells);
- protectors of delicate organs and other tissues against mechanical damage – think of a lamb kidney surrounded by its dense coat of suet;
- providers of palatability, flavour and texture and thereby enhancing the attraction and enjoyment of food.
- Current teaching that saturated fat causes heart disease is completely wrong. There is absolutely no evidence to support it.

Fat as a fuel

Most of the energy at low levels of physical activity is derived from the mobilisation of free fatty acids. At high levels of activity, contribution is made from carbohydrate stored as glycogen in the muscles and converted by them to glucose for their exclusive use.

Workers engaged in heavy physical activities, such as mining, forestry etc. seem to function well and remain fit on a diet in which fats contribute up to 40% of energy, provided that the fat intake does not exceed energy expenditure.

At extreme levels of strenuous, sustained physical activity, demanding more than 80% of maximum oxygen uptake (e.g. athletic competitions), carbohydrate is used almost exclusively. This basically unnatural activity requires a low fat/high carbohydrate diet; the carbohydrate being refined, energy-dense, high-calorie in type, requiring expert supervision. Remember that in our ancestral diet the carbohydrates were of the highly complex form found mainly in leafy vegetables and constituting the major part of a diet high in nutrients, but of low energy density. At such extreme levels of exertion, the glycogen stores in the muscles are sufficient for no more than two hours. Thereafter, the blood sugar falls dramatically (hypoglycaemia) with a fall in efficiency and a rising demand for free fatty acids (which in many leaned-down athletes are lacking).

Protein is almost never used directly by muscle for energy. Certainly, where consumption is above daily requirement, the excess can be converted to carbohydrate and so used for energy purposes; at the worst, further converted to fat. Conversely, starvation, when other sources of fuel are lacking, can lead to body proteins being broken down to maintain some function; mainly of the brain and nerve tissue.

Favourable levels of dietary fat

Provided that adequate daily physical activity[1] is being maintained, all the evidence so far indicates that levels of total fat intake of 25 to 30% of daily energy requirement approach the ideal. In those developed countries where the intake is greater, some reduction is essential. Equally in those societies where, perhaps because of poverty, lack of availability or ignorance, intake is lower, steps should be taken to increase levels. In each case, the aim should be the provision of a proper intake of

[1] See Exercise, pages 141-145

Components of food
More about Fats

essential fatty acids in correct proportions (i.e. 2:1 or 1:1 omega 6 and omega 3 – in the brain, the ratio is 1:1) and their derivatives; the long chain polyunsaturated fatty acids, eicosapentaenoic acid 20:5, n3, docosahexaenoic acid 22:6, n3 and arachidonic acid 20:4, n6. (refer to pp 76 & 77).

The "ideal ratio" between omega 3 and omega 6 fatty acids can vary greatly between individuals. The total requirement of both is raised in conditions of stress and disease.

The proportional requirement for omega 3 rises in colder, higher latitudes where sunshine is less.

Suffice it to say that the current ratio in Britain of around 14:1 omega 6 to omega 3 is grossly unbalanced.

The pregnant mother, the mother breast-feeding her baby, the growing child[1], all have extra needs.

To give you some ideas of how to estimate the quantities and types of fat in the food, refer to Guidelines – quantities pages 218 & 219.

---

[1] See Nutrition for the Family – Mother and baby, pages 150-156.

Fats – Chemistry
Components of food

The next few pages of simple chemical descriptions are intended to help towards a better understanding of some of the different fats and their roles.
If you have no knowledge of, or interest in chemistry (or, maybe are sufficiently well-informed as to find it *too* simple), ignore this section and go straight to Carbohydrates on Page 79.

Fats are, in chemical terms very simple substances. They are essentially chains of carbon atoms to which the other atoms are attached.

Carbon has the ability to link to four other atoms at one time, (tetravalence) eg. the gas methane, where carbon is joined to four hydrogen atoms CH_4

All the links are occupied and the compound

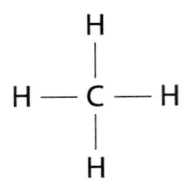

$$\begin{array}{c} H \\ | \\ H - C - H \\ | \\ H \end{array}$$

is said to be saturated and fairly stable.

A saturated fat, such as stearic acid would have eighteen carbon atoms

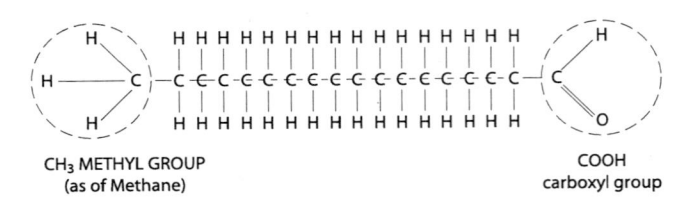

CH₃ METHYL GROUP (as of Methane)   COOH carboxyl group

COOH (carboxyl group) turns it into an acid, hence 'fatty acid'.

The body makes use of a number of saturated fatty acids.

1   Short-chain saturated fatty acids, such as butyric acid with four carbon atoms and caproic acid with six. These are used mainly for energy by the intestinal flora (bacteria).

2   Medium-chain saturated fatty acids include caprylic, capric and lauric acids with six, ten and twelve carbon atoms respectively. They are used mainly by the body for energy production and are not stored as fat.

3   Long-chain saturated fatty acids take part with polyunsaturated fatty acids (see below) in the formation of cell membranes. They tend to be solid at body temperature. Abnormally, they crystallise to form droplets which deposit in arterial linings. They also influence platelet[1] aggregation (stickiness) associated with clot formation and the resulting dangers of coronary heart disease, strokes and deep vein thrombosis.

Another type of linkage is possible, such as the gas ethylene C_2H_2, where two of the links are between the carbon atoms; a double bond.

We say that this compound is unsaturated;

$$H - C = C - H$$

chemically unstable and very reactive.

An unsaturated fat, such as olive oil with a single double bond, is called mono-unsaturated. It has eighteen carbon atoms, with a double bond at the ninth carbon atom.

Oleic acid (olive oil)

CH₃   9   COOH
18:1 *n*9

The Essential Fatty Acids (EFAs)

Essential fatty acids by strict definition are those that cannot be made in the body, but have to come in the food we eat. They are **Linoleic acid**, derived mainly from vegetable sources and **alpha-linolenic acid** derived mainly from animal sources.

---

[1] platelets: tiny blood cells essential to the mechanism involving blood clotting. They are important in preventing blood loss and for the sealing of any wound following injury.

Fats – Chemistry
Components of food

Linoleic acid has eighteen carbon atoms and two double bonds at the sixth and ninth carbon atom (18:2 *n*6)[1]

Linoleic acid

Linolenic acid has eighteen carbon atoms and three double bonds at the third, sixth and ninth carbon atoms (18:3 *n*3)

Linolenic acid

Fatty acids sharing two or more double bonds are termed *polyunsaturated*

Animals can insert double bonds

Animals, including humans, cannot synthesise the essential fatty acids, nor insert double bonds in *n*-6 and *n*-3 positions. they can however, introduce further double bonds between the originals and the carboxyl group

They can, additionally, lengthen the chain to twenty and twenty two carbon atoms to form long chain fatty acids of the loosely termed essential[2]; three of the most important are arachidonic acid - AA - (20:4 *n*-6) Eicosapentaenoic acid - EPA - (20:5 *n* 3) and docosahexaenoic acid - DHA - (22:6 *n*-3) The one, AA, vitally important in the development of the brain of the fetus during pregnancy and of the infant after birth and in the formation and elaboration of the cardiovascular system and the others, EPA and DHA, are two of the most important essential fatty acids involved in the structure and function of the brain and neural system.

Given these essential fatty acids, the body can further elaborate them by combination with various proteins, phosphorus, sulphur, to form other lipids used for other structural or functional purposes. As I have mentioned before, over 60% of your brain and mine and nerve tissue are composed of lipids. All cell membranes are made of lipid material as are many hormones as well as the materials that transport minerals and other essentials around the body.

---

[1] *Fatty acid formulae are abbreviated in the form x:y, n-m where x = number of carbon atoms, y = number of double bonds and m = the position of the first double bond measured from the methyl end. Sometimes n - m is omitted where the position of the first double bond is not known or a group of isomers (of similar structure but varying positions of the double bond/s) is represented.*

[2] *Some people lack the enzymes to do this and would of necessity have to derive them "ready made" in the foods they eat.*

Fats – Chemistry
Components of food

Trans fatty acids

Most naturally occurring isomers have what is termed *cis* configuration, giving the molecule a particular shape which allows it to attach itself to a particular place in or on the cell.

Because the nature of the double bond is unstable, polyunsaturated fats are inherently fragile and easily damaged. Exposure to light, air (oxygen) or heat can cause distortion or "twisting" of the molecule, producing the *trans* configuration.

cis fatty acid

$$CH_3(CH_2)_7\underset{H}{\overset{H}{C}}=\underset{(CH_2)_7COOH}{\overset{H}{C}}$$

trans fatty acid

$$CH_3(CH_2)_7\underset{H}{\overset{H}{C}}=\underset{H}{\overset{(CH_2)_7COOH}{C}}$$

Although the chemical composition is similar, the physical shape and, therefore, the biological effect is different. The lipid can no longer "fit" into its allotted place: akin to a bent key's jamming in a lock and rendering it inoperable – even worse, preventing the use of an undamaged key.

In my opinion, because of the malfunctions they cause, trans fatty acids (unlike saturated fats) are dangerous. Where possible avoid them.

They are known to interfere with lipoprotein metabolism[1] therefore increasing the risk of cardiovascular disease, of exacerbating inflammatory bowel disorder (Crohn's, ulcerative colitis), auto immune disease, e.g. rheumatoid arthritis and increasing the risk of breast cancer.

Trans fatty acids are to be found in all "spreads" and butter substitutes as well as in vegetable cooking oils such as corn (maize), safflower, sunflower, rape oils; also in commercial salad dressings, mayonnaise, potato crisps (chips, USA), fried foods, cakes, biscuits and in most restaurant foods where oils other than olive oil are used.

The basic structure of the main groups of the fats

Starting from Glycerol (Glycerine)

Triglyceride

$$\begin{array}{c} H \\ | \\ H-C^1-OH \\ | \\ H-C^2-OH \\ | \\ H-C^3-OH \\ | \\ H \end{array}$$

$$\begin{array}{c} H \\ | \\ H-C^1-OOCR^1 \\ | \\ H-C^2-OOCR^2 \\ | \\ H-C^3-OOCR^3 \\ | \\ H \end{array}$$

---

[1] see section on Cholesterol, pages 81-82

Fats – Chemistry and Carbohydrates
Components of food

Phospholipid
(example: choline phosphoglyceride - lecithin)

$$\begin{array}{l} H-C^1OOCR^1 \\ H-C^2-OOCR^2 \\ H-C^3-O-P(=O)(O^-)-OCH_2CH_2-N(CH_3)_3 \end{array}$$

(phosphorus)

R^1, R^2, R^3 represent similar or different fatty acids. Positions 1 and 3 in the carbon chain are usually occupied by a saturated fatty acid and position 2 by one that is unsaturated.

Carbohydrates

Carbohydrates are essentially a source of energy and, in this regard, as important as fat.

Carbohydrates are so-called because they are basically a combination of carbon (C) and water (H_2O). One of the simpler sugars is glucose $C_6H_{12}O_6$.

The word carbohydrate can be used to denote any kind of carbohydrate, or a mixture, or one in particular.

Carbohydrates are most abundant in seeds of the grass family, the graminae, which includes wheat, barley, oats, rice, rye, millet and maize. They occur in root vegetables, the pulses such as beans, peas and lentils, but also, in more complex form, in green leafy vegetables. As we saw when discussing protein, there is also a small amount in meat and fish.

Like proteins, carbohydrates are often large molecules made up from hundreds of simpler units, in this case simple sugars (monosaccharides). They can be divided into two main categories:

Indigestible carbohydrates, mostly cellulose and lignin (woody material) found in vegetables. Although not digestible by ourselves, they can be utilised by bacteria which inhabit mainly the large intestine to produce vitamins and vitamin-like substances, which we need. There, bacteria also work to provide the bulk – so called fibre – to ensure correct transit of material through the digestive tract.

Digestible Carbohydrates of which there are three types.

The first and largest is starch. This is derived mainly from grains (cereals), root vegetables and pulses.

The second and, these days, increasingly large group is composed of sugars. Sucrose – common table sugar – is derived from sugar cane and sugar beet. Lactose, is a sugar found exclusively in milk.

The smallest group consists of glucose and fructose, two of the simplest sugars and occurring mainly in fruits of different kinds.

The ultimate effect of digestion of carbohydrate is to produce a fuel; mainly glucose.

Digestion of starch begins in the mouth. An enzyme (a digestive chemical called ptyalin) breaks it down to a smaller molecule called maltose, which is further broken down to the smaller unit; glucose. This is why, if you chew a piece of bread or potato and hold it in your mouth, you will soon detect a sweet taste.

Sucrose is broken down rapidly in the stomach into glucose and fructose.

Lactose is broken down in the small intestine to glucose and another simple sugar, galactose; the latter being turned rapidly into glucose.

These sugars are absorbed from the digestive tract, mainly in the form of glucose and transported by a special blood supply directly to the liver, where some is stored in a more compact form, glycogen or

Carbohydrates
Components of food

animal starch. At this time, the pancreas – a gland with several different functions – releases a powerful hormone, insulin, which sensitises muscles to assimilate the circulating glucose and convert it into glycogen for their own use.

This is how things should work (and do) if the carbohydrates present are in the very complex form found in leafy vegetables, most tubers, roots and berries. These foods which are rich in micro nutrients, have a low energy/calorie value and conform to those eaten by our early ancestors and to which, over hundreds of thousands of years, our bodies are adapted. Because the digestion of these foods and the absorption of their contents proceed relatively slowly, blood sugar levels remain at a comfortable norm; neither rising nor sinking excessively.

Things have changed during the past 12,000 or so years.

Today, most of the carbohydrates eaten are in the form of starches derived from grains, some tubers such as potato and increasing amounts of sugars; mainly sucrose and fructose. They have a high energy/calorie content (but low nutrient value) and are very rapidly absorbed, with the consequence of high levels of blood sugar (hyperglycaemia) and increased insulin levels (hyperinsulinaemia). Because of the body's loss of control of sugar levels they can swing from very high to very low (hypoglycaemia) accompanied by feelings of weakness, drowsiness, sweating and craving for sugar.

Here follows a mad merry-go-round.

Excess sugar which cannot be stored as glycogen is converted to fat, leading to fat deposition, weight gain and obesity; excess circulating fats and high levels of insulin prompt the body to increase production of cholesterol while, at the same time, the tissues become less responsive to the high insulin levels (insulin resistance); decreased removal of glucose from the blood means that sugar levels remain high; the constant high levels of glucose and insulin cause damage, not only to the heart and major blood vessels, but also to the very fine vessels feeding the extremities (feet and hands) and those in the eyes and brain. This is why many sufferers from diabetes may be inflicted with gangrene – especially of the feet and toes – and with blindness.

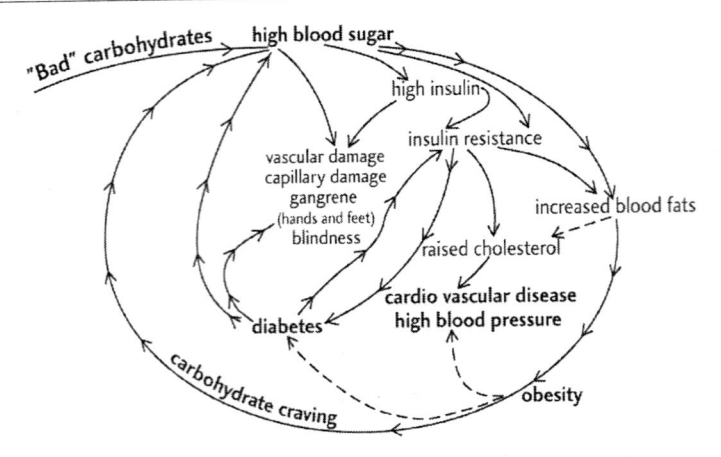

"Good" carbohydrates and "Bad" carbohydrates: The Glycaemic Index GI

Until the early part of the 20th century, it was not recognised that carbohydrates vary considerably in composition and in their effect on the health of the consumer. While some confer benefit, other constitute a danger – leading in particular to weight gain, obesity, heart disease, diabetes and many other ills.

The obvious need for a means of distinguishing that which is beneficial from that which is harmful sparked-off investigations to produce the *Glycaemic Index*. This is a measure of the rate and extent of rise of the blood sugar after the ingestion of a standard amount of a particular carbohydrate or carbohydrate-containing food: the frame of reference is that of glucose, set at 100. The index is the product of observations of groups of presumably healthy volunteers over the past 20 years, listing

Carbohydrates and Cholesterol
Components of food

hundreds of different items. Because human beings are not identical, so individual figures in any test differ and the result is not a precise figure but an average. Nevertheless it provides a very useful practical working guide.

Arbitrarily, figures of 65 and above are labelled "bad", between 35 and 65 "borderline" and below 35 "favourable" or "good". Needless to say, leafy vegetables, most roots and tubers, fungi and berries – to which our bodies are best attuned – have the most favourable ratings. *(For a list of examples, see Guidelines, Glycaemic Index page 222)*.

Cholesterol

Although, nowadays, seeming to have evil connotations, cholesterol is a normal, important constituent, not an intruder. Between 70% and 80% is made in the body; mainly in the liver and the intestinal mucous membrane. It is the most commonly occurring steroid and is found in most living organisms, although not in plants.

Cholesterol is a hard, waxy, fatty substance essential for our health. It is manufactured in the body from acetates (vinegars) from the breakdown of sugars and starches. It is also made from some fats, but not essential fatty acids and, exceptionally, from protein.

The Cholesterol Molecule

Cholesterol is required:

- as an integral part in the structure of all membranes and is vital as a regulator of the fluidity/flexibility of membranes, so maintaining their optimum functions;

- for brain and nerve function: synapses (connections between nerve cells) depend almost entirely on cholesterol.

- for the formation of circulating lipo-proteins (the agents used for transporting fats in the blood);

- as a precursor of steroid hormones[1] and vitamin D (from sunlight);

- as a precursor of the bile acids produced in the liver;

- secreted by skin glands, protects against dehydration, maintains flexibility and protects from damage by radiation, impact and infection.

Cholesterol is to be found in all tissues, all membranes, the nerve sheaths (myelin), central nervous system and is vital to hormone production.

Dietary cholesterol is found only in foods of animal origin; moderate amounts in meat and fish, more in offals, such as liver, kidney, heart and most in eggs and shellfish.

Surprisingly, a high intake of dietary cholesterol has little influence on the total amount circulating in the blood, as has been shown by much research done over many years. A diet rich in saturated fats will not cause cholesterol levels to rise.

Current "received wisdom", which is being constantly and uncritically parroted, dictates that acceptable levels of total cholesterol should lie between 3-5 mmol/L – the lower the better. This is inspite of repeated researches showing that lower levels (<3 mmol/L) are associated with increased depression, suicides and other serious mental disorders while higher levels up to 7.5 mmol/L do not appear to present any danger.

---

[1] *Steroid hormones include those produced by the cortex (outer part) of the adrenal glands, the gonads (ovaries and testes) and the placenta.*

Cholesterol and Fibre
Components of food

Several lipoproteins (fat/protein compounds), manufactured in the liver and in the digestive tract, act as *transporters* of cholesterol. Strictly speaking, they are not fractions of cholesterol, but two are used to denote total amounts:

- Low density lipoprotein, LDL, (ideally less than 3.3 mmol/L) conveys cholesterol to the cells and arterial walls: the absence of antioxidants, especially vitamin E, can result in fatty deposits (see notes on atherosclerosis).

- High density lipoprotein, HDL, (ideally more than 1.2 mmol/L) can remove atheromatous deposits from arterial walls and convey cholesterol to the liver for elimination.

From this you can see why, in the past, LDLs have been labelled as 'bad' cholesterol and HDLs as 'good' cholesterol. This is wrong, as both have essential roles; each being complementary to the other. It is when they are out of balance that problems arise.

Cholesterol levels can be made to rise by excess intake of sugar and of starches, which are readily turned, by digestion, into sugar and thence to fat.

Equally, high levels of cholesterol can be reduced by increasing the dietary levels of essential fatty acids; notably the omega 3 group, derived mostly from the sea foods. Physical activity and exercise, of which more later, are powerful factors for restoring balance.

Fibre

Originally called roughage, fibre was believed to be found only in vegetables and to consist of indigestible materials (mostly from cereal brans) such as cellulose, hemicellulose and lignin. It was thought to provide "bulk" to assist passage of food through the intestine, creating the image of a sort of intestinal loofah; certainly not my idea of fun to have an abrasive working its way along the delicate lining of my digestive tract!

In fact, fibre is a technical term. Certainly, many of its components are not digestible by ourselves, but can be broken down by the several hundred different species of (mostly friendly thank Goodness!) bacteria that inhabit our insides; approximately 1.5 kg ($3-3^{1}/_{2}$ lbs) of them. In the process, these bacteria produce vitamins (e.g. vitamin K) and vitamin-like substances for our benefit, while at the same time they proliferate, so increasing the bulk of the bowel content, rendering it softer and reducing the transit time – speeding the rate at which food passes along the gut. The effect is also to increase the frequency and ease of bowel motions. You see, the greater part of the stool that we pass consists not so much of food residue, as many believe, but of dead bacteria.

Prebiotics

These are substances in food, mostly vegetable, which we cannot digest or assimilate and can be classified as fibre. Some are insoluble, as in the fibrous or woody parts of plants and some are soluble. They can, however, be broken down by bacteria, the bowel flora, which inhabit the large intestine (colon) to provide their nourishment.

A healthy human digestive tract is host to approximately 1.5kg ($3^{1}/_{2}$ lbs) weight of estimated

Fibre
Components of food

to be one thousand different species of bacteria; mostly friendly. Two of the best known beneficial species include many strains of Lactobacilli and Bifidobacteria. They help to reduce colonisation by opportunistic, unfriendly bacteria and yeasts by producing their own antibiotic substances. They also produce short-chain fatty acids like acetates and butyrates which the cells lining the intestine can use for fuel. Additionally others produce B vitamins and vitamin K, participate in the control of cholesterol levels and maintain the integrity of the intestinal lining.

Sources of prebiotics, oligosaccharides, are in most vegetables. Of the common vegetables, the richest are the lily family – onions, leeks and shallots. Tubers of Jerusalem artichoke are particularly well supplied; too much for some people who find the oligosaccharide content overstimulating, causing excessive intestinal gas. Other good sources are in roots such as salsify and scorzonera.

Although most fibre comes from vegetable sources such as leafy greens, roots, fruits and berries as well as brans, there is some in most meats and fish[1]. Even that famous black stout from Ireland, Guinness, contains fibre in the form of soluble pentose sugars that we cannot use, but some of our intestinal inhabitants can (not that I recommend it as one's main source!).

Lack of fibre is linked to many disorders; notably constipation and resultant haemorrhoids associated with inco-ordinate gut movement (peristalsis) and straining to evacuate a hard stool; diverticulosis – a consequence of increased pressures generated in attempting to move along the unnaturally small and hard gut contents. Inflammation of the resultant pockets formed, results in the painful, sometimes dangerous, condition of diverticulitis. Colon cancer is linked to inadequate fibre. The consequent stagnation leads to the accumulation of toxins, of which the prolonged contact with the lining of the bowel can lead to the development of cancer.

A diet high in fibre, as eaten by people in Africa, is said to be the reason for their very low levels of coronary disease as compared with those in the Western societies. I am not convinced. There are many other factors; consumption of sugar and refined starches for instance, being much less among African people. Certainly, they have very low levels of intestinal disorders, such as appendicitis, diverticulitis and colon cancer. On the other hand, an excessive amount of fibre in the diet, as occurs in some African communities who consume very large quantities of plantain (a type of coarse cooking banana), can result in the painful and dangerous condition of volvulus. This is where the intestine twists on itself – an excruciatingly painful event – thereby cutting off the local blood supply. If not relieved promptly this leads to gangrene of the affected part and death.

Today, we are being constantly urged to increase our fibre intake by eating, especially, whole-grain cereals, with their bran coating, or bran itself. How can this advice be correct?
- If cereals only appeared in man's diet a few thousand years ago . . .
- If none of us is equipped to deal with raw starch in any quantity . . .
- If constipation and all the ills that follow; appendicitis, diverticulitis, colon cancer are all diseases of civilisation . . .

How did our ancestors survive and thrive through the millions of years before us? I hope that by now you will have worked out some of the answers. . .

---

[1] In the early 1950's, Professor Hugh Sinclair noted that the Inuit (Eskimo) people had no plant food during most of the year. He surmised that unabsorbed animal mucopolysaccharides were performing the role of fibre as in other pure carnivores.

Water

Not a food as we understand it, water is, nevertheless, a nutrient of the highest order.

Of your total bodyweight and mine, nearly three quarters is water. The proportion in our brains is similar and, believe it or not, water comprises almost a quarter of the weight of our bones.

Although most of us can survive for many weeks without food, we can run short of water within days. Unlike most animals, Man is very profligate with water, having no special mechanism for conserving it. It is lost, not only through the kidneys as urine and the skin as sweat, but also through the lungs (themselves almost 90% water) as vapour. Physical activity increases the loss in proportion to the effort and can vary from two litres (two quarts) in twenty four hours to over four times that amount during strenuous activity.

Replenishment can take many forms; water, soups, beverages (such as tea, coffee, tisanes). All foods supply water, especially leafy vegetables and fruits. During the process of combustion of food for energy purposes, water is also produced as a by-product, so that even if some people seem to be sparing of their intake of liquids, it is probable that they can stay in fluid balance so long as their energy expenditure remains low.

A word of warning

"Drink two to three litres of water daily" is advice currently given to people living relatively sedentary lives. "Drink as much water as possible" has been the advice given to athletes, especially cyclists and marathon runners. Excess of water intake during exercise can cause a fall of sodium levels in the blood. Seven deaths and over two hundred and fifty casualties have occurred in athletes during the past forty years.

The answer: drink only to satisfy the thirst experienced, but no more.

Ideally the water we drink should be clean and pure.

During the nineteenth century in England, the introduction of filtered, cleaned and chlorinated water on tap was hailed as a great advance. Together with the new closed system for sewage disposal, it proved to be the most powerful single factor in reducing illnesses and deaths caused by contaminated drinking water. All the developed countries have followed suit with great benefit; one not yet shared by a very large proportion of the world's less privileged people.

Municipal water supplies are derived from various sources; deep bore-holes, rivers, reservoirs and reclaimed water from water treatment plants. It has been said that London (UK) water has been recycled through the human body at least six times before it is drawn from the tap. True or not, this and other fears have prompted many people to buy extremely expensive bottled "pure" or "natural" waters in ignorance of the fact that the majority are derived from the same water as is supplied to their homes. The difference lies in the fact that the bottled water (often in plastic, which can leach harmful solvents) has been filtered through charcoal to remove any possible unpleasant taste, but without removing any of the many soluble contaminants that may be present. These include oestrogens, which some authorities consider to be a factor (among many others) responsible for the increase in breast cancer in women.

What was not known when chlorination of drinking water was first introduced, is that chlorine reacts chemically with some of the soluble organic substances in the water to produce potentially dangerous compounds. One group, *trihalomethanes*, known to be carcinogenic, may, together with other risk factors such as tobacco smoking, influence the development of cancers of the bladder, colon and rectum.

Aluminium salts are also added, at water treatment plants, to precipitate solids (rather similar to the fining of beers and certain wines to clarify them). Aluminium is, however, a toxic element which can produce neurological damage and has been associated with some cases of brain dysfunction[1]. Aluminium salts are not removed by filtration.

Although the quality of most municipal water supplies is better than ever before, the sheer cost of eliminating all contaminants, nowadays amounting to thousands and *of which most are man-made*, is prohibitive. Consequently, many people, especially in the USA, have begun to install water purifying systems in the home. The best, water-distillation by steam, will produce water with as little as 10 parts per million of contaminants compared with the public water supply varying from 300 - 1000 parts per million. Another system, reverse osmosis, is expensive and requires more maintenance, but provides clean water to 20-40 parts per million.

Natural water from rivers, springs, wells and bore-holes cannot now be relied upon for purity. In recent decades, man-made contaminants have increased in numbers and amount. Effluents from factories, rubbish in landfill sites, farm waste and fertilisers have been seeping into rivers and ground water. Airborne chemicals, mostly from industry and power stations, falling as rain, have been detected even in the High Andes and Himalayas. In some parts of the world, notably the USA and India, many people have died or been made seriously ill by *naturally occurring* arsenic poisoning local well water.

All is not gloom, however. Even if you cannot afford a steam distiller or a reverse osmosis unit, remember that Man is amazingly resilient and adaptable. *Our bodies are equipped to survive.*

Provide the necessities:

- adequate sleep;

- adopt appropriate exercise for your type;

- use and *maintain* **the simple principles of good nutrition as I have already described;**

- **love God and your neighbour and drink water!**

Your system will do the rest.

---

[1] "Disturbance of cerebral function by aluminium in haemodialysis patients without overt aluminium toxicity." Altman P. et al. Lancet 1989; 2:7-12

Chapter 6

Free Radicals and Antioxidants

Free Radicals and Antioxidants

It seems to me that the generally held view is that antioxidants are "good" and that free radicals are "bad" (just as the components of cholesterol, HDL and LDL are often described). This is far from the truth. Each group is as necessary as the other.

Free Radicals

Free radicals are elements produced in the body and are only dangerous when uncontrolled. They are crucially important in the immune functions and the many other chemical reactions taking place. These include the placing of oxygen in precise amounts where it is needed for energy production within the body cells.

Oxygen in excess is destructive and free radicals are extremely energetic (and by design, self-perpetuating – see panel) so that unless carefully monitored and controlled, runaway reactions result in severe damage and subsequent death.

There are also external triggers of free radical activity. They include radiation (sunlight, x-rays, radon gas), tobacco smoke[1] and other air pollutants from factories and vehicle exhausts, man-made herbicides and pesticides and the abundance of artificial additives that have invaded the food chain. Excessive physical effort also causes a rise in free radical activity.

Just as polyunsaturated fats in the body can be damaged by unchecked free radical activity, so can those found in certain vegetable oils be affected when exposed to light, air (oxygen) and high temperatures. These oils when fresh (e.g. cold-pressed linseed, sunflower and maize) are often described as "sweet" meaning pleasant and acceptable to taste. Because of their chemical instability, these oils are readily oxidised by free radicals (lipid peroxidation) and become rancid – rank in smell and taste – instinctively repellent.

An atom of stable matter has pairs of electrons spinning around the nucleus. When an electron in the outer shell is lost, the atom becomes a free radical – electromagnetically unbalanced. It now behaves like a magnet and, to restore its stability, grabs an electron from the nearest neighbour so creating another free radical and setting up a chain reaction which, if uncontrolled, produces a cascade of damaging free radical activity.

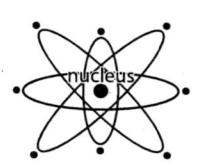

a stable atom surrounded by paired electrons

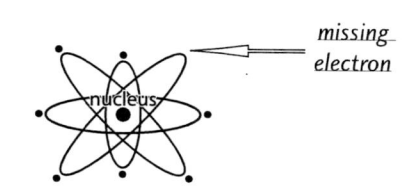

an unstable atom with an unpaired electron in the outer shell becomes a free radical (missing electron)

---

[1] *Some years ago, the British Medical Journal printed a number of photographs of which 50% were smokers. Viewers were invited to identify the smokers, on appearance only.*
Most were identified by the increased wrinkling of the skin; evidence that smoking had caused an increase in free radical damage, with destruction of the elastic tissue.

Free Radicals and Antioxidants

These *trans* fatty acids (see the section on Fats-chemistry) are particularly dangerous. They are commonly present in manufactured foods but their presence may be masked by other stronger flavours present. They can be detected when these foods or oils are heated – who hasn't experienced the rank smell of overheated oil outside many eating places?

Illustration courtesy Bev Williams

Never eat healthy food

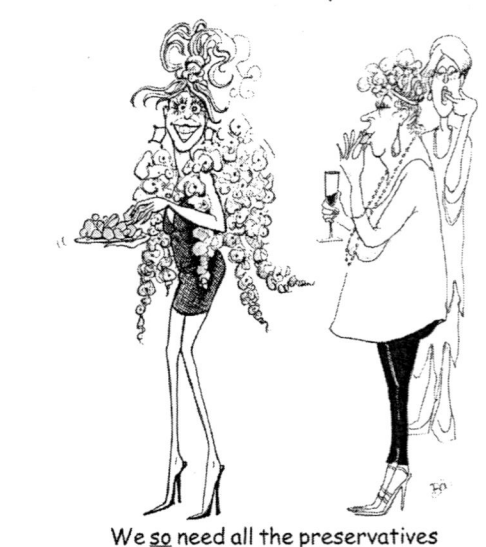

We *so* need all the preservatives we can get.

Antioxidants

Antioxidants match the free radicals in numbers and variety. They are found in all living matter. We have them (thank God!) in all the tissues and inside every cell in our bodies. Inside the cells, some protect the membranes, some protect the mitochondria (energy producers) and others prevent damage to the nucleus and its contained DNA, which holds the entire genetic code of each one of us.

Most antioxidants come in the food we eat; the great majority from *fresh* vegetables and fruits. Others are obtained in animal foods and some are manufactured in the body.

Vegetable sources provide:

- trace minerals including copper, iron, manganese, selenium, sulphur and zinc;
- vitamins including the carotenes (vegetable precursors of vitamin A), B_1, B_2 and B_6, C (including the flavonoids), E complex and K;
- Antho and proanthocyanadins.

All are present in various forms in the leaves and roots of different vegetables, including the fungi (mushrooms). Carotenoids are present in all dark green leafy vegetables as well as in red and yellow coloured fruits, vegetables and flowers. Flavonoids, in company with vitamin C[1], abound in the skins of coloured berries such as blackcurrant, blueberry, cranberry, haw from hawthorn and black grapes.

The fat soluble vitamin E complex found in various seeds and nuts, prevents oxidative damage (rancidity) in polyunsaturated fats; not only in plants but also in our bodies *(see panel page 93)*. Many other oils with strong, specific antioxidative activity exist in herbs such as rosemary, thyme, oregano and basil and in spices that include cinnamon, cloves, coriander, cumin and turmeric, among many others: a good reason to *invigorate*, in more senses than one, food for the family by the judicious and regular use of herbs and spices.

---

[1] Unlike the artificial form prepared from glucose, vitamin C in nature is never "pure". It is always accompanied by other antioxidants, usually flavonoids, with which it works in synergy. Purified vitamin C, on its own, can work as an oxidant (free radical).

Free Radicals and Antioxidants

Animal sources provide:
- vitamin A, all the Bs, D, E and K;
- trace elements as found in plants, but usually in more bio-available form;
- Ubiquinone, Co Enzyme Q_{10};
- glutathione, a tripeptide and powerful antioxidant and, like vitamin C, a detoxifier;
- essential fatty acids, notably but not exclusively, from oily fish and shellfish. Usually, all are more richly supplied in offal meats; less so in muscle meat.

Antioxidants made in the body include:
- vitamins A (from carotenes when needed), D (in the skin from the conversion of cholesterol by ultra-violet radiation in sunlight), all the Bs and K (by the bowel flora);
- Co Enzyme Q_{10};
- glutathione and its analogue, alpha-lipoic acid;
- Melatonin – a hormone and very powerful antioxidant manufactured by the pineal gland; part of the brain.

Unfortunately for most of us, production of glutathione, Co Enzyme Q_{10} and Melatonin goes downhill from about the age of 50. Even more unfortunately there has been in Britain at least, an even more marked reduction in the consumption of offal meats – the richest sources. Add to this the fact that we in the UK are eating much less of fresh vegetables and fruits than 50 years ago and that there has been in that time, a progressive decline in the mineral contents of all, except marine, foods.

For these many reasons availability of antioxidants and the protection they provide has diminished. It is no wonder that despite greater affluence, illnesses suggestive of faulty metabolism have been increasing: cancers, cardiovascular diseases, mental disorders, infertility, diabetes, osteoporosis, autoimmune conditions such as rheumatoid arthritis, allergies – to name but a few.

Gloomy? Take heart . . . . . all is not lost!

Firstly, we must choose our food very carefully. Look back to food (pages 39-59). Secondly, because the quality of food – mineral and vitamin content, for example – has been declining steadily, however carefully you choose to eat there is the likelihood of some deficiency. Which means that some sort of judicious supplementation would be appropriate.

None of this would have been a problem to our early ancestors of, say, 200,000 years ago, even if their life-expectancy was almost certainly shorter due to the hazards of the environment and the fact that the people of that time were at the bottom of the "learning curve". (Today, we have the advantage of millions of man-years of gathered knowledge and experience.) Population pressures were small and food was abundant in quantity, variety and quality. Wild foods – even today – are richer in mineral and vitamin content than their cultivated cousins. Additionally, the foods on offer were those to which Man's chemistry had adjusted during the previous four million or so years of his evolution.

Free Radicals and Antioxidants

Supplementation

If we are to consider supplementation, let us first remember some of the facts:

- Bigger is not better. The body likes balance not great quantity;
- vitamin A, vital for life, in large amounts is toxic. Even relatively moderate amounts (10,000 i.u. daily) in early pregnancy have been associated with birth defects;
- B vitamins in food do not come singly, except for B_{12}. Early experiments showed that an excess of B_1, produced a relative deficiency of B_2. B_6 in sustained high dosage (above 300-400mg) can, in some people, cause nerve damage and mood change – fortunately reversible on reduction of intake;
- vitamin C in Nature is never alone, but accompanied by other antioxidants and behaves like an antioxidant and detoxifier (purifier). In the pure form it can reverse its role, becoming an oxidant;
- the carotenes never appear singly, but in groups. Beta carotene is cited as being biologically the most active, but on its own *and in the absence of vitamin C* can, in certain circumstances, become harmful. In fact it is known that people who smoke and who supplement with beta carotene, have an *increased* risk of developing lung cancer;
- vitamin D, like vitamin A absolutely necessary for life, also becomes toxic in excess, causing excessive deposition of calcium, not only in bone but in soft tissues including the blood vessels, tendons and kidneys.

Nor do the metallic elements escape:

- Iron as it occurs naturally in food does not cause the digestive upsets that occur with forms commonly available from pharmacies;
- Magnesium in food causes no problems but in artificial preparations can behave as a stomachic irritant, an antacid or a laxative but not be assimilated;
- Chromium, an essential element in the control of blood sugar levels, is in some supplemental preparations, carcinogenic: yet not as it appears in food.

These are just a very few examples. Before rushing off to the health food shop:

1. Refer to the sections of vitamins and minerals. There you will find food sources and, additionally, some idea of your daily requirement.
2. Select a reliable supplier of good quality, safe supplements;
3. If possible, seek the help of a professional nutritionist – they do exist;
4. Ideally, at least initially, undertake a laboratory analysis[1] in collaboration with your nutritional advisor, to obtain values for your own levels of vitamins, minerals, antioxidants and essential

---

[1] In the UK we are blessed with the capabilities of THE BIOLAB MEDICAL UNIT, 9 Weymouth Street, London. Telephone +44 (0)20 7636 5959/5960

Free Radicals and Antioxidants

fatty acids and their combinations known as cholesterol esters;

5 Be prepared to be patient. We may live in the age of instant coffee, but remember that we are living creatures. Adopting the correct pattern of eating and using any necessary supplementation will not produce instant results.

Certainly some improvements may be noticed within a few weeks but changes for the better will continue for many months and in some chronic conditions, years. Be assured that they *will* occur to produce a state of increased, prolonged well-being and capability.

How antioxidants work

Just as antioxidants do not come singly in foods, but in hundreds, so they do not operate singly in the body, but in groups.

Here is a simple example:

An unsaturated fat (lipid) having lost an electron becomes a free radical but can be rescued by vitamin E which donates one electron. Vitamin E minus its electron is itself a free radical. It can in turn be restored by a carotenoid's donating an electron.

Last in the chain, vitamin C, with its attendant bioflavonoids, by sacrificing an electron rescues the carotenoid. Vitamin C has now become a radical but, unlike the others, is stable and, therefore, harmless and can safely be voided in the urine.

$$\begin{array}{l} \text{lipid } ^{-e} \\ \quad \downarrow \longleftarrow \text{vitamin E } ^{+e} \\ \text{lipid } ^{+e} \\ \quad \downarrow \qquad\qquad \text{vitamin E } ^{-e} \\ \text{carotenoid } ^{+e} \longrightarrow \downarrow \\ \quad \downarrow \qquad\qquad \text{vitamin E } ^{+e} \\ \text{carotenoid } ^{-e} \\ \quad \downarrow \longleftarrow \text{vitamin C } ^{+e} \\ \text{carotenoid } ^{+E} \\ \qquad\qquad\quad \text{vitamin C } ^{-e} \\ \qquad\qquad \text{excreted in urine} \end{array}$$

From this you can see how important it is that there must be an adequate amount of each antioxidant at every level, but with particular attention to the last – vitamin C – the detoxifier.

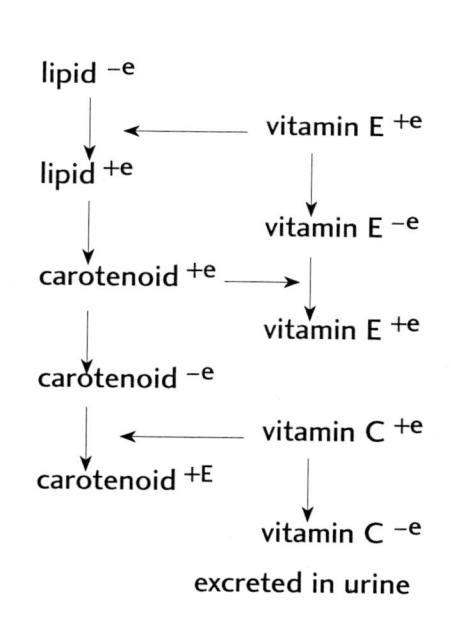

Chapter 7

Vitamins

The Vital Amines
Casimir Funk (1884-1967)

Kazimierz Funk was a Polish biochemist who pioneered research into vitamins. Born in Warsaw, he studied in Berlin and then in Bern, Switzerland where, in 1904, he gained a doctorate in organic chemistry. He then went to work at the Pasteur Institute in Paris, once more in Berlin and then at the Lister Institute in London.

In 1915, he went to America where, in 1920, he became a naturalised citizen. He returned to his native Poland in 1923, but found the existing political turmoil unsettling so, in 1927, left for Paris to found his own institution, the Casa Biochemica.

During his time in Europe, Funk had read of the work of Christian Eijkman, a Dutchman who had observed that people who ate brown rice were less liable to suffer from beri-beri than those who ate fully refined rice. In 1911, Funk established that middlings (the coarse discard from milling) from rice could cure beri-beri in pigeons. These extracts contained nitrogenous substances called amines and so he surmised, incorrectly, that he had discovered a new class: *vital amines* or *vitamines*. Later knowledge revealed that not all vitamins were nitrogen-containing amines and so the "e" was dropped.

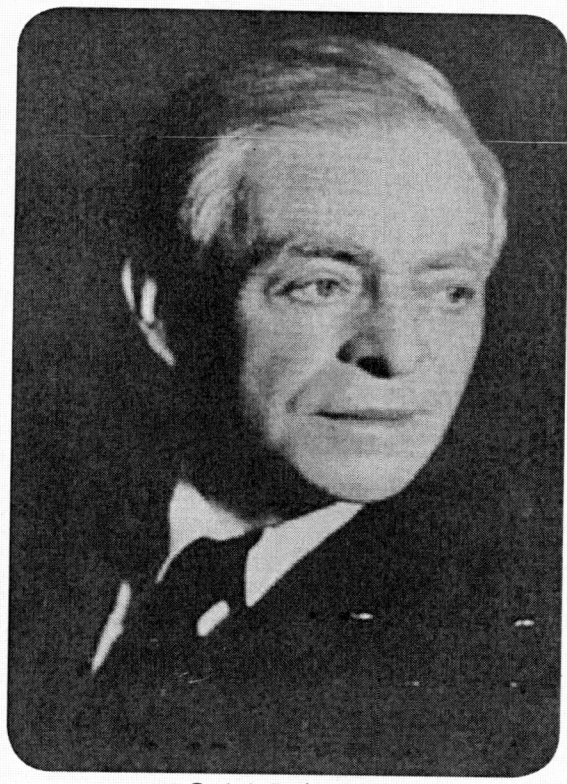

Casimir Funk at 70

Nevertheless, Funk was the first to isolate nicotinic acid (niacin, vitamin B_3) and subsequently to postulate the existence of other nutrients essential to health (viz. vitamins B_1, B_2, C and D).

At the outbreak of War in 1939 and following the German invasion of France, Funk returned to America and, in 1940, inaugurated the Funk Foundation for Medical Research. Here he did extensive research into hormones and the biochemistry of diabetes, ulcers and cancer. He also pioneered improvements in commercial drug production and developed several commercial products of his own.

Dr Casimir Funk died in New York in 1967, aged 83.

Vitamins

Vitamins do not form part of body structure, but without them, none of the body chemistry would work.
They can be magical in restoring health, preventing illness and even death.
Vitamins alone do not, however, turn a bad diet into a good one.

This section is basically a synopsis of what we know about vitamins (remember, they were only identified during the early part of the twentieth century) and the role of each as it forms part of the food we eat.

> **It is not meant to be a plan for self medication; ideally supplementation should only follow laboratory measurement and be applied by trained professionals.**

Preface to Vitamins

Oxygen is a ferociously active and destructive gas, yet is essential for the life of oxygen breathing creatures. In the course of evolution these creatures, including ourselves, developed many protective mechanisms to cope with this poison.

Similarly, what we now call vitamins originated as toxins developed by plants for self protection against animals[1]. In the course of evolution the animals first developed detoxifying mechanisms, but later used the toxins or their derivatives for their own benefit.

The Vitamins

In the main, vitamins are substances that are not made in the body, but have to come in the food we eat. Although they do not form part of the structure, without vitamins none of the body chemistry would function.

Their effects can be spectacular when even minute amounts can not only prevent illness but cure; even prevent death.

Make no mistake! If you take vitamins in the belief that, miraculously, you will achieve good health while on nutritionally poor diet, you will be disappointed (and out of pocket). Besides, in my opinion – I say this with some circumspection, although I have researched this carefully over many years – we in the UK have probably only *one* really reliable producer of nutritional supplements out of dozens; in the USA, only *four* out of hundreds.

Let us consider each one in turn and ask the following questions:

1. What does the vitamin do?
2. In what foods do you find it?
3. What are the effects of deficiency?
4. Can it be harmful?

---

[1] *Rabbits are able to thrive on some plants e.g. belladonna which are poisonous to other animals. Deer can consume considerable amounts of bracken, lethal to other species. Koala bears' sole food, eucalyptus leaves, are full of poisons. In contrast, there is a variety of dhal (lentil) used extensively in parts of India as food. Unlike others, it contains poisons which can cause illness and death; yet because of ignorance and pressure from landowners, is still being cultivated and eaten.*

The Vitamins

Vitamin A (Retinol) and Beta carotene

Vitamin A (Retinol):

This is a fat soluble vitamin and, like all vitamins has multiple functions.

Vitamin A is needed:

- for the developing fetus and the infant and is involved in the development of the cardio vascular system and of the smooth muscle of the arteries;
- for the proliferation and migration of the cells in the brain and nervous system;
- for the development of the pancreas and of the cells that produce insulin. (It is thought that the lack of Vitamin A at the time of development may be one of the causes of diabetes);
- for the protection against cancer;
- for healthy eyesight, particularly for night vision;
- for normal bone development and growth;
- for reproduction; synthesis of sex hormones;
- for health of skin and mucous membranes;.
- for its potent immune function and antioxidant activity.

Sources

The richest sources are liver and fish liver oils. Beta carotene, derived from vegetable sources such as carrots and dark green leafy vegetables, is a precursor of vitamin A (i.e. it can be converted to vitamin A if there is a deficiency). It is destroyed by cooking at high temperatures.

Deficiency of vitamin A affects vision. It is associated with night blindness and with blindness in deprived children. It is also one of the factors linked to infertility in men and in women. It is also associated with breakdown and poor healing of skin and mucous membranes, lowered vitality and increased susceptibility to infection.

In excess, vitamin A is toxic. It gives rise to dizziness, intense headaches, nausea and vomiting: in extreme cases, cirrhosis of the liver. Like other fat soluble vitamins, it is stored and, if intake is excessive, levels can rise dangerously. A daily intake, in the adult, of 4,500 mcgRE (micrograms of retinol equivalent), or approximately 15,000 I.U. (international units), is considered generally to be safe. In a child, under 13 years, suitable intake should be approximately one sixth of the adult dose.

Beta carotene is a natural vitamin A precursor, water soluble and widely distributed in fruits and vegetables. It forms part of their orange and yellow pigment and derives its name from carrots; one of the richest sources. It is destroyed by cooking at high temperatures.

Beta carotene is only one of a family of over five hundred different carotenoids found in various coloured fruits and vegetables; each having slightly different protective functions.

The Vitamins

Beta carotene – The B Vitamins

Beta carotene:

- has powerful antioxidant and free radical activity;
- has ability to improve night vision;
- assists in protection of the cardiovascular system;
- is reported to improve skin tone and, through its anti free-radical activity, protects against ageing.

Deficiency of Beta carotene is associated with failure of the immune system and, where there is accompanying lack of vitamin A from animal sources, symptoms of vitamin A deficiency.

A word of caution: recent research has associated Beta carotene intake with *increased* incidence of lung cancer among cigarette smokers. The mechanism is not yet fully understood.

Because Beta carotene is converted to vitamin A only as the body requires it and any excess is excreted in faeces, or stored in the body cells, it is considered non-toxic. Excess may show as yellowing of the skin and sweat.

Preface
The B Vitamins

These are water soluble vitamins and although we shall be considering them singly, remember that, with one or two exceptions, nature offers them to us as a group. In other words, they operate in balance. Because they are water soluble, they tend to enter and leave the body rapidly and require daily replenishment.

The Vitamins

Vitamin B_1 (Thiamine) – Vitamin B_2 (Riboflavin)

Vitamin B_1 (Thiamine):

- helps to maintain the proper function of the nervous system;
- helps to maintain normal energy activity and assists in the mechanism of carbohydrate metabolism;
- is needed for the normal function of muscle and the heart;
- is necessary for normal growth and development;
- helps to maintain the health of mucous membranes.

Sources

Sources of vitamin B_1 are to be found in the cells of all meats, poultry, the pulses (peas, beans, lentils) and whole grains. In foods that are boiled, loss occurs **a** by heat and **b** by leaching into the water.

Deficiency of vitamin B_1 can lead to Beriberi; more commonly to polyneuritis, heart and circulatory disorders, lack of growth, muscular weakness and emotional imbalance.

Vitamin B deficiency also occurs in chronic alcoholism as a result of increased requirement of the vitamin and because many alcoholics have a very inadequate diet. This can lead to polyneuropathy and to a condition known as Korsakow's syndrome: an amnesic state in which the inability to record new memories leads to confabulation and to the paradoxical situation in which the sufferer can carry out complex tests learned before his illness (like driving a motor car) but cannot learn the simplest of new skills.

Vitamin B_1 appears to be non-toxic in amounts of 500mg or more per day. Except in cases where there is a measured deficiency, or very high physical activity, a sensible daily upper limit would be around 100mg.

Vitamin B_2 (Riboflavin):

- is necessary to enable the release of energy to be derived from food. Vitamin B_2 requirement increases in line with physical activity, pregnancy and breast feeding;
- with vitamin B_1, it is important in maintaining the proper functions of the nervous system;
- like vitamin B_1, it helps to maintain the health of mucous membranes;
- is necessary for proper brain function, whether increased mental activity, or in conditions of stress;
- aids normal growth and development and integrity of the joint tissues;
- may be critical in maintaining fertility.

Sources

Sources of vitamin B_2 include meat, especially liver and other offals, poultry, fish, nuts, whole grains, eggs and green leafy vegetables. It is less sensitive to heat than vitamin B_1, but can be destroyed by exposure to light.

Deficiency is associated with polyneuritis, poor mental function, gastrointestinal disorders and skin problems.

There seems to be no toxicity associated with B_2. Any amount in excess of the body's needs is spilled over into the urine imparting a bright yellow-green colouration.

The Vitamins

Vitamin B_3 (niacin, niacinamide)

Vitamin B_3 (niacin, niacinamide):

This vitamin comes in two forms; Niacin, or nicotinic acid and a combined form Niacinamide; each with slightly different actions.

Vitamin B_3:

- is involved with energy production. It is an essential component of a mechanism known as the Kreb's cycle (tricarboxylic acid cycle: citric acid cycle) allowing for intermediates derived from fat, carbohydrate or amino acids to be completely oxidised (burnt) to carbon dioxide and water by the mitochondria (energy components) in the body cells: for energy production and in tissue repair. The requirement rises in line with physical activity;
- is needed for the health of nervous and digestive systems;
- improves circulation by dilating blood vessels (Niacin);
- can improve tinnitus (ringing in the ears) and dizziness;
- is involved with the mechanism of the blood sugar control and therefore, useful in avoidance of, or in the treatment of, diabetes;
- is effective (Niacin) in the treatment of some forms of schizophrenia.

Sources

Sources of vitamin B_3 are meat, poultry, seeds, nuts and fish.

Deficiency is associated with a disease called Pellagra[1], difficult to assess because B_3 is involved in so many different activities. We can infer that low levels are associated with diminished physical capability and stamina, poor circulation and impaired mental ability.

Toxicity is generally considered to be low, but Niacin (nicotinic acid), in doses above 30mg, can cause intense flushing with uncomfortable burning and itching of the skin. In addition, incautious use can cause gastritis (inflammation of the stomach) for some people.

Unlike vitamins B_1 and B_2 which are heat sensitive and so are reduced in amount by prolonged cooking, B_3 is remarkably heat stable.

---

[1] Pellagra means rough skin. Exposed skin becomes rough and dark. Other effects are diarrhoea and mental upsets, including irritability and depression. Untreated pellagra can be fatal: hence referred to as the disease of the four d's; dermatitis, diarrhoea, dementia and death.

The Vitamins

Vitamin B$_5$ (Pantothenic acid) and Vitamin B$_6$ (Pyridoxine)

Vitamin B$_5$ (Pantothenic acid)

This vitamin is largely concentrated in the brain. Like other vitamins, it has many functions.

Vitamin B$_5$:

- is required for proper brain development and activity, in combination with other nutrients;
- is involved with formation of neuro transmitters (chemicals involved in correct function of brain and nerve tissue);
- is involved in manufacture of body fuels; glucose and fatty acids;
- is essential for the correct function of the adrenal glands and for the manufacture of the steroid hormones, including "stress hormones" and vitamin D;
- Requirement is raised by increase of mental and well as physical activity.

Sources

Sources of vitamin B$_5$ are wide spread and include meat, liver, poultry, fish, egg yolk, pulses, seeds, some fruits (such as oranges and tomatoes) and green vegetables.

Deficiency is difficult to identify, except by inference. Athletes, having their B$_5$ status measured, and given appropriate supplementation improved their performance; implying that their levels had previously been below optimum.

Toxicity has not been established. Doses of up to 10 grams daily for several weeks produced no observable ill effects, with the exception of one or two cases of loose bowels and water retention.

Vitamin B$_6$ (Pyridoxine)

This vitamin is known as a 'helper'. It functions as a coenzyme (helper) at every level of protein metabolism as well as that of fat and sugar.

Vitamin B$_6$:

- is involved in the making of haemoglobin for new red blood cells and all new proteins;
- helps to make essential brain chemicals;
- helps to make enzymes for the metabolism of essential fatty acids, also for the burning of glycogen (animal starch) in energy production;
- is involved in maintaining fluid balance;
- is necessary for the defence system, producing antibodies;
- helps in the conversion of the amino acid tryptophan (from the digestion of protein) to form niacin (vitamin B$_3$);
- is needed to aid the absorption of vitamin B$_{12}$;
- has been used successfully in the treatment of some forms of depression and schizophrenia.

The Vitamins

Vitamin B$_6$ (Pyridoxine) and Biotin B$_8$

Sources

Sources of vitamin B$_6$ are liver, meat, egg yolk, some fish, pulses, nuts and seeds.

Deficiency of vitamin B$_6$, because of the range of its activities, can be seen in many different forms; depression and other psychological disorders, anaemia, water retention, lowered energy and stamina, skin disorders and (in conjunction with zinc deficiency) brittle nails and hair loss.

Toxicity is generally low and, as has been pointed out in relation to water soluble vitamins, daily supply is necessary. High doses, in excess of 300-400 mg can, for some people, produce neuropathy; mostly numbness and tingling sensations in hands and feet and loss of co-ordination. This effect is reversible by lowering the dosage. High doses are, in any case, unwise because they cause rapid depletion of the body's glycogen store, with consequent loss of stamina.

Biotin B$_8$

This vitamin takes part in the formation of three different enzyme systems: one for the generation of glucose, another for the formation of new fatty acids – both major fuels – and the third for the break down of certain amino acids, for the synthesis of of new protein.

Sources

Good sources of Biotin are liver, egg yolk, oily fish (herring, mackerel, pilchard, sardine, tuna, salmon) soya and brown rice. Biotin is also synthesised by friendly bacteria, which inhabit the healthy intestine; the bowel flora. It is heat stable.

Effects of deficiency are difficult to identify as, even in the poorest diets, Biotin is always present. It is thought that low levels may be associated with some forms of skin trouble, falling hair and muscular weakness.

Biotin has no known toxicity.

The Vitamins

Vitamin B_9 Folic Acid (Folate, Folacin)

Vitamin B_9 Folic Acid (Folate, Folacin)

This is another helper substance of the B vitamin group. Known as a co-factor, it is a complex family of substances.

Folic Acid:

- is essential for reproduction and the growth of cells, especially red blood cells;
- is essential for the normal function of the nervous system. In the developing fetus, is required for the proper construction of the brain and spinal cord and is, therefore, a most important requirement before and during pregnancy;
- helps proper cell growth in the digestive tract;
- helps regulation of histamine levels in the body, affecting both the antibody reactions and mental stability;
- is involved in the fundamentals of protein synthesis.

Sources

Sources of Folic acid are liver, egg yolk, fresh dark green leafy vegetables and legumes. Folic acid is easily destroyed by heat, exposure to light and to prolonged storage at temperatures above 8°C (48°F).

In the developing fetus, deficiency of Folic acid leads to malformation of the developing nervous system and is linked to the conditions of spina bifida (incomplete development of the spinal cord) and anencephaly (failure of brain development). Deficiency also inhibits new cell growth, especially those having a high turn over such as in muscle, red blood cells and cells of the gastrointestinal tract.

Toxicity of Folic acid is low. Although the daily requirement may be 400-800 mcg (millionths of a gram), experimental much greater supplementation has produced no observable ill-effect. A word of caution is needed here. Excess of Folic acid, when there is a deficiency of vitamin B_{12} may mask the signs of pernicious anaemia – a potentially fatal disorder.

Equally, if vitamin B_{12} levels are low, addition of folic acid can unmask (or precipitate) a serious neurological condition know as subacute combined degeneration of the spinal cord.

The Vitamins

Vitamin B_{12} (Hydroxocobalamin, Cyanocobalamin)

Vitamin B_{12} (Hydroxocobalamin, Cyanocobalamin)

Vitamin B_{12} is a family of substances, cobalamins, with the metal cobalt as base. It is required for the formation of all cells and, like folate, particularly for the high turnover cells as in bone marrow, red blood cells and cells in the gastrointestinal tract. It is involved in the synthesis of the insulating covering of the nerves, the myelin sheath and for energy production. Vitamin B_{12} is also essential for the correct working of the nervous system and for the metabolism of folic acid.

Sources

Of all the B vitamins, this is the only one to be derived solely from animal foods and not from vegetables. Meat, especially liver, eggs, shellfish, such as mussels and oysters, are all good sources. There are, however, some moulds or fungi which can produce the vitamin, which may explain why some people, living in parts of Asia, with little or no access to animal foods, rarely show signs of deficiency.

Deficiency of vitamin B_{12}, due to lack in the diet, is rare. It can occur in people on faddy diets and in vegans, (vegetarians who take no food that has animal associations; even milk and cheese). The consequence is of the development of a form of anaemia; the inability of the body to manufacture haemoglobin, the red oxygen carrying pigment in the blood. An accompanying deterioration in the nervous system occurs with numbness and 'pins and needles' in the feet and legs, weakness and a lack of balance in walking; also mental deterioration. Untreated, pernicious anaemia[1] is fatal.

Incredibly, the daily requirement, about one millionth of a gram, is so small that you would not be able to see it with an ordinary optical microscope. Yet, this is the amount that can mean the difference between total good health – and death.

There is no known toxicity from vitamin B_{12}. Amounts of many thousand times the daily requirement have been administered without any ill-effects.

---

[1] **Pernicious anaemia** *is an auto-immune condition caused by production of antibodies either to certain cells in the stomach or 'intrinsic factor' and so affecting absorption of vitamin B_{12} in the lower part of the small intestine.*

The Vitamins

Vitamin C (Ascorbic Acid, Ascorbates)

Vitamin C is essentially a water soluble vitamin, although there is also a fat soluble form, ascorbyl palmitate. It takes part in the formation of collagen; a protein involved in the structure of all connective tissue in the body, including skin, bones and joints. It is an important antioxidant (an 'anti rusting' agent preventing damage to tissues from the toxic effects of oxygen in excess; as iron, in the presence of moisture, is attacked by oxygen in the air to form rust). Other important functions of vitamin C are:

- to enhance immunity to infection;
- to form part of the mechanism of haemoglobin production;
- to act as a detoxifier.

Sources

Nearly all fresh leafy vegetables and most fruits are good sources of vitamin C. It is, however, a fragile substance and is easily destroyed by heat and prolonged storage. Citrus fruits, such as lemons and limes, are rich sources. Oranges, traditionally considered to be a good source, are unreliable and, because of varied methods of production, have sometimes been shown to contain none at all.

The effect of deficiency of vitamin C has been known for centuries. Scurvy, a dread disease, first affected those sailors attempting long sea voyages. It first manifests as laziness, low spirits and irritability, followed later by easy bruising and bleeding – especially of the gums, which become soft and spongy. Later, teeth would loosen and fall out, skin blotches would appear where bleeding had occurred and haemorrhaging into the joints would cause crippling pain. In the early eighteenth century, Dr James Lind, a naval surgeon, learned that fresh oranges and lemons could prevent or cure the disease, as could fresh vegetables and other fruits. In 1753, he published a book 'A Treatise of the Scurvy' with his observations. Forty years later, the Royal Navy began to adopt Dr Lind's findings – issuing lime juice (lemons were originally called limes) as part of the ration for the next two hundred years. British sailors were, therefore, known to Americans as Limeys; a term which nowadays seems to apply to all of us in Britain[1]. Other less dramatic effects of vitamin C deficiency are increased proneness to infection, iron deficiency anaemia and premature ageing of skin and joints.

Vitamin C is considered to be non-toxic. Because man, like primates and guinea pigs, cannot make vitamin C, it has to come from food. Nearly all other animals can manufacture vitamin C and do not suffer from a lack in their diet. Estimates of the daily requirement vary greatly. About 30mg daily will prevent scurvy, but it is considered, by researchers, that for optimum health, a daily intake of between 1,000 and 2,000 mg is more realistic. Good nutrition should supply, at least 1,500mg daily. Because our individual chemistry varies widely, tolerance to large doses differ, but can give rise to abdominal colic and diarrhoea.

---

[1] *As, at that time, limes were rare and expensive, poorer folk – especially in winter – derived vitamin C from onions. There is a story of a sailor's being flogged, in the 18th century, for stealing onions from the ship's stores, which were low after a prolonged voyage.*

The Vitamins

Vitamin D (Calciferol, Cholecalciferol)

Vitamin D (Calciferol, Cholecalciferol)

D consists of a group of fat-soluble substances called calciferols. Despite its name, it may not be a true vitamin but is most certainly a steroid hormone of supreme importance. Because every cell in the body requires calcium in order to function correctly, vitamin D is essential. During pregnancy, vitamin D is vital for the correct development of the brain of the growing fetus. Epidemiological evidence links the lack of this rather neglected vitamin to being one of the factors leading to the occurrence of schizophrenia in later life. (Pregnant mothers should not, however, take extra vitamin D without proper professional assessment and advice.)

Vitamin D:

- "makes strong bones" by regulating absorption and use of calcium and phosphorus (both constituents of bone) thereby increasing bone density;
- assists in the assimilation of vitamin A from the diet;
- works synergistically with vitamins A and E in the formation of protective enzymes of the immune systems;
- is essential for the growth and maturation of the white blood cells – also part of the body's immune defences;
- stimulates pancreatic production of insulin;
- reduces polyps in the colon and inhibits growth of pre-malignant cells in the colonic mucous membranes;
- exhibits plurality of anticarcinogenic activity.

Sources

Vitamin D is to be found in fish liver oils (notably cod and halibut), in the livers of other animals and in small amounts in eggs. Most importantly, it is also formed when ultra violet light in sunlight reacts on the cholesterol in human skin. The vitamin from these sources is also known as vitamin D_3. It is converted by the liver and kidneys to the active form; I alpha cholecalciferol. Skin pigmentation in people living in countries such as Britain with relatively low levels of sunlight can prevent such production and result in deficiency of vitamin D. The vitamin can also be produced artificially by irradiating certain foods that contain a different steroid called ergosterol, with ultra violet light to form vitamin D_2 – calciferol. This latter is frequently used to 'fortify' some items such as margarine or baby-foods.

In children, when vitamin D deficiency is present, the bones tend to be soft and become distorted and malformed; the condition is known as rickets. In the adult, because all the body cells demand calcium and as the bones are a convenient store, calcium is taken from the bones for other purposes. This is one of the factors leading to the condition of osteomalacia and its attendant dangers.

Because vitamin D is fat soluble, any excess cannot be excreted in the urine and so can accumulate to toxic levels. These give rise to loss of appetite, vomiting, irritability and depression.

The Vitamins

Vitamin D (Calciferol, Cholecalciferol) *continued* and Vitamin E (Tocopherol)

Children can become comatose and even die. Long term excess can result in deposits of calcium in the soft tissues – commonly the linings of the blood vessels leading to occlusion, and of the kidney with the formation of calculi (stones).

The current recommended daily allowance (RDA), 10mcg=400i.u. errs on the side of caution. Many authorities consider that it should be set much higher – perhaps to 50mcg=2,000i.u.

Certainly many people in the UK risk deficiency and require a higher intake.

They include:

- dark skinned people living in areas of low sunlight intensity;
- night workers;
- people living or working mostly indoors;
- women who are pregnant, or who are breast-feeding;
- vegans;
- people whose work, or culture, requires them to be fully clothed at all times;
- most people during the winter months – October to March, inclusive (in the Northern Hemisphere and, no doubt in the corresponding Southern latitudes).

Vitamin E (Tocopherol)

This is, in fact, a family known as tocopherols. These are fat soluble and have different functions. The vitamin we are considering here is d-alpha tocopherol. Before it was properly identified, it became known as 'the sex vitamin' because when experimental rats were deprived of it, the females were able to conceive, but the offspring died in the womb and were reabsorbed, while the males eventually became sterile. Other animals deprived of vitamin E show different ill-effects. For us humans, vitamin E acts as an antioxidant to prevent deterioration, or rancidity, of body fats, notably the essential fatty acids and any other unsaturated fats which by their nature are easily damaged. In conjunction with the mineral selenium, vitamin E is involved in the formation of protective enzymes.

Sources

The tocopherols are found in leafy green vegetables, in vegetable oils and seed oils *(where they act as a natural preservative)* cereals, eggs and animal foods.

Effects of deficiency are diverse. Unlike vitamin B_{12} lack which can be associated with pernicious anaemia, or vitamin D deficiency with rickets, vitamin E acts, together with other nutrients, in a much wider field. Lack of it can, therefore, be associated with heart and circulatory disorders, malfunction of the immune system, some forms of diabetes and other medical conditions. It is easily destroyed by food processing. As consumption of processed food is increasing, there may well be a general shortage in the population.

Toxicity is considered to be very low, but there have been occasional reports of raised blood pressure in doses higher than 1,200 units daily.

The Vitamins

Vitamin K (Phylloquinone) and Other Substances

Vitamin K (Phylloquinone)

This fat soluble vitamin of which there are several forms, is important for the formation of prothrombin, which is one of the substances that enable the blood to clot. It is also involved in the formation of two of the structural proteins in bone and so influencing its strength. Comparatively little research has been done on vitamin K, but recent information suggests that it is one of the body's anti-cancer agents; either causing aberrant cells to revert to normal function or causing them to destroy themselves (apoptosis).

Sources

In the diet, fresh green leafy vegetables provide the best source. The friendly bowel flora that inhabit the healthy intestine also manufacture vitamin K.

Because vitamin K is manufactured in the gut, it is most unlikely for you to suffer any deficiency under normal conditions if eating correctly.

It can, however, decrease in certain disease states, such as obstruction of the bile duct. This would prevent bile salts, essential for absorption of fats and fat soluble vitamins, from reaching the digestive tract. The result would be spontaneous haemorrhaging into tissues (bruising) and joints, excessive bleeding from even light injury and spontaneous nose bleeds. Severe liver disease is also associated with depleted levels of vitamin K.

Many hospitals routinely give injection of vitamin K to babies at birth to prevent haemorrhagic disease of the newborn.

The current recommended daily requirement of 80mcg. is almost certainly an underestimate. A healthy and varied intake of dark green leafy organically grown vegetables, ensuring a hale and hearty bowel flora would supply at least twice this amount.

There is no recorded toxicity to vitamin K.

Other Substances

Sometimes called vitamins, but not truly so because they can be made in the body.

Inositol (Cyclohexane hexol)

Is a simple naturally occurring sugar-alcohol with many functions.

Inositol:

- increases the action of brain neurotransmitters, such as serotonin and noradrenaline and so acts as a stress reliever to lower anxiety levels – calming without lessening mental alertness;
- restores diminished insulin sensitivity to liver and muscle as well as improving the function of the insulin-producing beta cells of the pancreas; so helping to lower raised blood sugar levels;
- improves protein synthesis of skeletal muscle as well as muscular tissue of heart and intestine; so diminishing the tendency for the muscular loss associated with aging;
- is important for the maintenance of all cell membranes and, therefore, for the efficient function of all the cells in the body;
- reduces some forms of addictive behaviour.

The Vitamins

Inositol (Cyclohexane hexol) PQQ and CoQ10

Sources

Inositol is widely available in foods of animal origin, fish, meat and offals, as well as from vegetables, pulses and fresh fruit. It is also manufactured in the healthy kidney from circulating blood glucose as well as by the friendly intestinal bacteria.

In theory, there should be no deficiency of Inositol in the diet. A functional deficiency may be present if there is insufficiency or imbalance of the essential fatty acids, or in a diet rich in sugar, starches and/or saturated fat.

The effects of such a deficiency would be widespread including anxiety states, depression, chronic fatigue syndrome, bowel disorder, diabetes.

The daily requirement is not known and none has as yet been recommended.

There is no known toxicity to Inositol.

Choline is used in the manufacture of cell membranes and the brain neurotransmitter acetylcholine.

Pyrolloquinolone quinone PQQ,

is important for the formation of collagen; to maintain health of skin and all connective tissues: may be a true vitamin.

Ubiquinone (Co-enzyme Q10, CoQ10)

Ubiquinone (CoQ10) belongs to a family of substances called quinones. Ubiquinone, as its name implies, is ubiquitous – found everywhere. It is found in all human cells, with the highest concentrations in those which are most metabolically active: brain; liver; heart; kidneys and pancreas.

One of the body's natural chemicals, CoQ10 is plentiful in youth, but production declines with age.

CoQ10:

- is essential for the proper function of the mitochondria (energy components) in the cells;
- is necessary for the production of adenosine triphosphate (ATP), the fuel for all cells and body processes;
- is a very powerful antioxidant working in synergy with vitamin E to prevent damage to cell membranes from free-radical activity;
- activates macrophages, the "killer" white blood cells of the immune system.

Sources

Because CoQ10 is essential for the proper working of the mitochondria and, hence, energy production it is found in all cells, human, animal and plant.

The best food sources are offals, oily fish, lean meats, nuts and seeds.

Deficiency occurs when the diet is lacking the best food sources and with advancing age. This results in a deterioration of brain function and an increase in heart disease and cancer. Food sources alone cannot compensate for the insufficiency caused by the decline of the body's production of CoQ10. Supplementation, from the age of 50 years and onwards would seem to be justified: in the region of 50mg daily.

There is no known toxicity.

The Vitamins

Betaine and the Homocysteine Cycle

Betaine

- Betaine is a "methyl group" donor. *(See Chemistry of fats, pages 72 – 76).*

Like the recognised vitamins, it cannot be made by the body and has to come in the food we eat. On that basis, I think that it should also be regarded as a vitamin.

Other methyl group donors are choline, methionine and the vitamins B6, B12 and folic acid; all are involved in the homocysteine Cycle (see box).

The methyl group donors, of which Betaine is the principal, are needed for the formation and creation of:

- RNA and DNA;
- creatine and carnitine *(part of energy production)*;
- materials forming part of the body's defence systems;
- adrenal stress hormones, epinephrine and norepinephrine;
- phospholipids, for the manufacture of nerve tissue and cell membranes;
- neurotransmitters, controlling brain and nerve functions;
- controlling levels of the amino acid, homocysteine – high levels of which are associated with an increased risk of heart disease.

Sources

Vegetables of the beet family (chenopodiaceae) including edible wild plants or "weeds'" such as Good King Henry (c. bonus-henricus), fat hen (c.alba) as well as the garden plant Swiss chard; also eggs and fresh-water crustaceans (crayfish, shrimp) and mussels.

Deficiency of the methyl groups in foods eaten today in the UK is increasingly common affecting all those functions listed above. Raised homocysteine levels increase the risk of cardio-vascular disease (and indeed, can be used to predict it). Faulty DNA production is a certain cause of oncogenesis (cancer causing).

There is no known toxicity.

The Homocysteine Cycle

Cycle diagram:
- s-adenosyl homocysteine — breaks down to form homocysteine
- now transformed into s-adenosyl homocysteine, release of methyl group
- s-adenosyl methionine
- homocysteine
- Dietary methyl groups (betaine, choline) — combine with homocysteine
- circulating vitamins B₆, B₁₂ and folic acid
- to form s-adenosyl methionine SAMe
- methionine — to form methionine
- addition of adenosine triphosphate - ATP (an "energy packet" formed from glycogen and triglyceride fats)
- to be used for RNA and DNA; creatine and carnitine (energy production); materials for the immune system; adrenal hormones; phospholipids; neurotransmitters

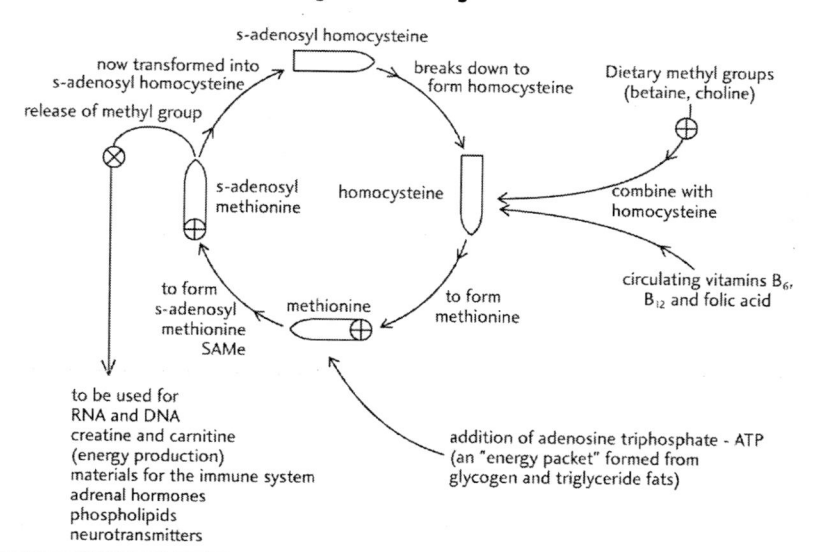

Deficiencies of the methyl groups in the diet are very common. This means that homocysteine formed from the breakdown of s-adenosyl homocysteine is not reconverted to methionine. The consequential high levels of homocysteine are toxic and are responsible not only for increased risk of cardiovascular disease, but also for damage to brain and spinal cord (together with deterioration of mental function) and other disorders involving muscles and joints.

Chapter 8

Minerals

Minerals

Introduction

Our bodies are made of minerals. They form part of the structure and, together with the vitamins, are involved in the myriad chemical processes relating to all physical and mental activities.

Each has not one but many different functions working not alone but together with many other substances to fulfil its role.

This section is intended to describe the individual minerals and the role of each as it forms part of the food we eat.

> **It is not meant to be a plan for self medication; ideally supplementation should only follow laboratory measurement and be applied by trained professionals.**

The Minerals

Before considering the minerals, understand that 95% of the total body weight is made up of five other major elements. Hydrogen and oxygen, mostly in the form of water (H_2O); carbon, which is the basic element in all organic matter ("organic chemistry" can be defined as the chemistry of carbon); nitrogen, the basic element in all proteins; sulphur, which is an element in many proteins. All are abundantly available in the air we breathe, the water we drink and the foods we consume.

Minerals form part of the body structure and, together with the vitamins, are crucial in the correct function of the body chemistry. Some, the macro minerals, are present in large amounts. Others, the trace minerals (micro nutrients) are present in minute amounts; thousandths or millionths of a gram. All should be present in the food we eat.

None works by itself, but in synergy with many other substances, including other minerals.

Carbon: a short note

This black, sooty substance is the element on which all life on our planet Earth depends and is the basis for the formation of all organic material.

Carbon is present in our atmosphere as a gas, carbon dioxide. It is absorbed and converted by plants to form their own structure. Animals cannot do this but, by consuming plants, can use the ready-formed organic material, altering it for their own needs. Some animals eat other animals, again making use of carbon containing material, so that there is never any risk of deficiency.

Carbon is abundant in all soil, having accumulated from dead and decayed vegetable and animal matter. It is returned to the atmosphere, in the form of carbon dioxide gas, by animal respiration (we expel it from our lungs as a waste product) and by the burning of wood and fossil fuels, such as coal, gas and petroleum products.

Sulphur

The reservoir of this macro-nutrient lies in the world's oceans. Through the activities of a species of phytoplankton, it is released into the atmosphere in the form of a benign gas, dimethyl sulphide, seeding clouds with sulphur, which falls in rain and is taken up by plants.

Minerals
Sulphur and Calcium

That is the good news.

The not-so-good news is that sulphur in the atmosphere can be harmful. When sulphur is burnt, a corrosive gas, sulphur dioxide, is formed. By interaction with water in the atmosphere it is turned into sulphuric acid which, when falling as "acid rain", is responsible for the destruction of vegetation and forests. Originally, nearly all sulphur dioxide came from natural sources; forest fires and, especially, erupting volcanoes which spew out large volumes of the gas.

Today, the problem is increasingly man-made. Most natural petroleum contains substantial amounts of sulphur. Attempts have been made during refining to reduce the amount in the lighter fractions, as used in motor vehicles. The very heavy remaining "sludge", with a consequently higher sulphur content is used in heavy industrial furnaces, power stations, iron and steelworks. Worst of all, marine engines in the thousands of vessels traversing the globe, using this heavy diesel fuel, produce more pollution world-wide than do the terrestrial sources. Hopefully, this is something that can be corrected.

In the body, sulphur is involved in the formation of the amino acids cysteine, cystine, methionine and taurine and, hence in the composition of many of the body's proteins: also the vitamins thiamine (B_1) and biotin.

Our daily requirement is large, approximately 1 gram, but easily obtained from the complete animal proteins (containing all the necessary amino acids), meat, fish, eggs and milk products. Proteins from vegetables tend to be incomplete and so mixing several, especially the legumes, peas, beans and lentils, is advisable. Onions and garlic are also good sources.

Calcium

Is the most abundant of the minerals, amounting to 1250 grams (not quite 3lbs) in a person weighing 70kgs (11 stone). Over 99% is in the bones and teeth. *The remaining 1% is necessary for the correct function of all the cells in the body.* Because of this constant need for calcium, bone acts, therefore, not only as the framework (skeleton) on which the body is built, but as a convenient place of storage for calcium. There are two groups of cells in bone; one group, the osteophytes (osteoblasts), extracts calcium that is circulating in the blood and uses it to form new bone; the other group, the osteoclasts, breaks down bone tissue to release calcium into the circulation. In other words, the calcium in the bone is not fixed but on the move. Hormonal influences are important in bone metabolism. They include those from the pituitary growth hormone (somatotrophin), the male hormone testosterone (present also in smaller quantities, in the female) progesterone and contributions from the adrenal glands: also parathyroid hormone and vitamin D. Bone is also plastic, that is to say it adjusts itself to the load imposed on it, becoming thicker and stronger in response to regular physical activity; this in addition to correct nutrition, of which more later.

Calcium is by far the most abundant mineral in bone, but the total content of minerals is only 50%; the rest consists of 25% water, 20% protein and 5% fat.

Minerals
Calcium

Calcium is necessary, not only for the formation of bones and teeth but for the correct function of nerves and muscles, including heart muscle. It is involved in proper function of the digestive system, absorption of vitamin B_{12}, control of iron, cholesterol and the blood clotting mechanism; not alone, but in conjunction with other elements in the food.

Sources

Calcium is present in a very wide range of foods. Although in different forms, they are equally well absorbed. It is available from all leafy vegetables and eggs, in moderate amounts; more so in seeds, nuts and pulses. Meat and offals supply calcium, but only in moderate amounts; more so in fish, especially canned fish, such as pilchard, sardine and salmon, where the bone has been cooked soft. Seaweeds of all kinds, samphire, shellfish, grains and milk products have much higher levels. Hard water can supply a substantial amount, perhaps 200mg of a daily requirement of 1000 mg.

Current advice, from the medical profession and every conceivable 'nutritional expert', is that, for bone strength, the source of calcium is from milk and milk products. Have you ever wondered from where the cow gets the calcium in the first place?

Horses bred in Ireland are sought all over the world. They are valued for their high quality, performance and strength of bone. They feed mainly on old permanent pastures.

These pastures consist of not one, but many different grasses and deep rooting 'weeds' and herbs. These provide an abundance not only of calcium, but of all other minerals and vital substances needed for the proper development of body and skeleton.

Deficiency in the growing child can result in rickets, digestive disorders, anaemia and poor development of the nervous system. In the adult, lack of calcium and other essential elements (also, other factors such as vitamin deficiency, lack of exercise, gastrointestinal upset leading to poor absorption) can give rise to osteoporosis, where calcium is leached from the bones, leading to weakness and possible fracture. A recent development, noted in America, has been that of osteoporosis in young women caused by the over-consumption of cola-type drinks. These contain phosphoric acid, upsetting the calcium/phosphorus balance and leading to calcium loss[1].

Phytates found in grains bind onto calcium rendering it insoluble, theoretically leading to deficiency. There is evidence, however, that man, unlike some other animals, can manufacture an enzyme to destroy phytate and so rendering the calcium available.

There is still no consensus about the daily requirement of calcium. Estimates vary between 500 mg to 1,200mg in the adult. The higher figure is probably more realistic.

Intake of calcium in excess of 2,500 mgs daily can lead to deposition of calcium in the linings of blood vessels, in the kidneys, with the formation of kidney stones, and interfere with the balanced interaction (synergy) with the other elements in the body.

---

[1] *Young men are protected from calcium loss, to some extent by the presence of relatively high levels of the male hormone, testosterone.*

Minerals

Calcium, Phosphorus and Magnesium

Phosphorus (Phosphate)

In the form of phosphate, phosphorus is the next most abundant mineral, about; 700-800 grams (1½ lbs) most of which, about 85%, is in the skeleton and is involved even more actively than calcium in body functions. It is necessary, with calcium for the formation of bones and teeth. Phosphate is an essential component of cell nuclei and of DNA, the genetic material in all cells. Phospholipids form part of virtually all cell membranes. It also enables efficient absorption of essentials in the food, energy production and cell reproduction.

Sources

Virtually every food contains phosphate. The average daily intake is probably around 1,500 mg, compared with 1,000mg of calcium. Deficiency is quite unknown.

In most circumstances, the body can deal very easily with too much phosphate. The exception is when phosphorus in artificial form is taken in excess, as mentioned with reference to cola-type drinks. Here, the excess phosphorus can displace calcium from bone and give rise to osteoporosis. Furthermore, increase of phosphorus relative to calcium is one of the factors involved with raised blood pressure and colon cancer.

Magnesium

This element, of which we have about 25-30 grams (1 oz), exists mostly inside the cells, 60% in bone. It is involved in more than 300 of the enzyme systems in the body, influencing physical and mental functions and exists in both water soluble and fat (lipid) soluble forms.

- It is vital for bone formation and assists absorption and retention of calcium.
- It is necessary for muscle and nerve function.
- It is needed for the utilisation of glucose as a fuel.
- It helps to maintain cardiovascular health and to regulate heart rhythm.
- It is one of the factors involved in transmission of the genetic code.
- It is involved in the mechanism of hormone production.
- It is now known to be a factor in the prevention of eclampsia and pre-eclampsia (toxaemia of pregnancy).

Sources

All meats and fish can supply magnesium in moderate amounts. Green leafy vegetables and legumes should be good sources, but can be deficient if grown with the use of artificial fertilisers, which cause an increase of water content and a reduction as well as imbalance of the mineral content of the plant. Refined cereal products have much of the magnesium removed and so-called "enriched" flours have not had the magnesium replaced. Daily requirements may vary between 300-400 mg. People who are physically active require more, as magnesium can be lost in the sweat. Like calcium, magnesium is present in hard water.

Because magnesium is involved with so many functions, the effects of deficiency are hard to identify clinically. Direct measurements of levels in serum (blood after the removal of the cells) and of levels inside the cells (intracellular) provide more reliable information.

Toxicity of magnesium in the organic form (as it would appear in food and copied in some food supplements) is low. Many inorganic forms can be very irritant to the gastrointestinal tract; others, such as magnesium hydroxide ("milk of magnesia"), magnesium sulphate (Epsom Salts) are not absorbed and are often used as laxatives.

Sodium

This element works mainly outside the cells. Combined with chlorine it becomes sodium chloride - common salt. Together with potassium and chloride it performs a host of electrical functions without which nothing in the body would work. These three elements are known as electrolytes; sodium and potassium being positively charged, are *cations*, while chloride, being negatively charged is an *anion*.

Sources

Sodium is present in all foods, more in animal products than in vegetables. While our daily requirement is probably only 1 gram (less than 1/30th of an ounce), so much is added to our food, whether by the manufacturer[1], or in cooking, or at the table, that the daily intake is often 10-15 times as much. It is interesting to note that herbivores will actively seek salt, whereas carnivores do not. Similarly, most people will add salt to foods of vegetable origin to improve palatability, but not to the same extent to meat or fish dishes.

In the United Kingdom, 80% of salt (sodium chloride) consumed comes from processed food. Bread accounts for one quarter. Sodium is also present in monosodium glutamate – so-called flavour enhancer – and in sodium bicarbonate, which is present in some processed foods and in some pharmaceutical indigestion preparations.

The body is so efficient at retaining electrolytes that extra sodium is not needed, even in very hot climates, or after strenuous exercise. You may think the opposite, because the sweat of most of us is salty. After prolonged sweating, however, the sweat becomes salt free and yet the body's sodium content remains constant.

Towards the end of the Second World War, I, with my unit, was transferred to India. After Europe, we all found the heat extreme and many of the troops suffered from an unpleasant form of dermatitis caused by excessive perspiration – sweat rash (prickly heat). We all dutifully took daily salt tablets to counter this; with no effect.

French troops in the tropics were not issued with salt tablets and did not suffer sweat rash. Each man, however, had a daily allowance of rough red wine; a good source of other minerals and antioxidants. There is a lesson here, somewhere!

Subsequent research by the British Army, in hot desert environments and by the Israelis, confirms that under such conditions, the body needs water, not salt.

---

[1] Hitherto, about one quarter of the salt consumed in the U.K. has come from bread. A recent report from the food standards agency in the U.K. indicates a move to reduce the amount of salt used in bread making and other manufactured products.

Minerals

Sodium, Potassium and Chloride

Excess salt (sodium) upsets the balance between sodium and potassium. This can give rise to water retention in the tissues and generalised swelling (oedema). Babies are very vulnerable to too much salt in the diet, because their kidneys are not able to excrete sufficient of the excess. In some adults, high salt intake is associated with high blood-pressure. It can also upset heart function by causing a relative loss of potassium, thus interfering with conduction of nerve impulses.

If salt is to be used in the home, I would recommend that sea-salt with its accompanying minerals in near-physiological balance be used as a safer alternative to rock salt (pure sodium chloride).

Potassium

This element functions mainly inside the cells. Together with sodium and chloride it is involved in the conduction of nerve impulses. We have about 250 grams in the body as potassium chloride.

- It is a co-factor (helper) in the formation and function of many enzymes.
- It helps to maintain fluid balance and acid/alkaline balance (pH).
- It plays a part in protein synthesis.
- It is part of the mechanism for detoxification and waste removal.

Sources

Sources of potassium are in all meats, fish, eggs, leafy green vegetables, grains, milk and fruit. It is interesting to note that Nature gives us potassium in relation to sodium in ratios varying from 3:1 in milk to 7:1 in fresh salmon. This accords to the diet on which Man has evolved. Unfortunately, our present diet, much of which is processed and to which salt (sodium) has been added, has reversed this to 2:1 in favour of sodium.

Because of the excess of sodium in the diet, it is possible to suffer a relative deficiency of potassium, which should not otherwise occur; there being a sufficiency in all fresh foods. The effects of such a relative deficiency would match those of an excess of sodium. Yet, in the absence of an excess of sodium the daily requirement of 3,500 mg of potassium would be easily met.

Potassium as it appears in food in its organic form is non-toxic.

Chloride (Chlorine)

This is the other half of common salt (sodium chloride) and is an *anion*, electrically negative, which works outside the cells. Together with sodium and potassium, it is necessary for the correct electrical functions, nerve conduction, fluid balance.

It is also necessary for the production of hydrochloric acid (HCl) in the stomach.

Because chloride is linked to sodium and because there is an excess in the modern diet, there is no likelihood of deficiency.

Toxicity is the same as that for excess of sodium.

Minerals
Chloride, Iron and Zinc

Iron

This element of which we have about 4 grams (about $1/7$ of an ounce) has many important functions.

- It is the essential component of haemoglobin, the protein in red blood cells which carries oxygen to all parts of the body. About half of the total amount of iron is in haemoglobin, about one third is in the bone marrow and the rest inside other cells, including as a component of myoglobin, (muscle pigment).
- It is important in the defence against infections. To any site of inflammation will be rushed a concentration of iron.
- It is a component of antioxidant enzymes to prevent lipid peroxidation (destruction of fat by oxygen) of cell membranes.
- It is needed for production of hydrochloric acid in the stomach.
- It is needed for the metabolism of B vitamins.

Iron is widely available in meats, eggs, vegetables and grains. The form of iron from meat, haem iron, is the best absorbed.

Considering its wide distribution, iron deficiency should be uncommon. The reverse is true. Firstly, the best source, haem iron, is only 10% bioavailable, while iron from other sources is only a mere 1%. Secondly, poor diet, lacking vegetables and meat and having a preponderance of refined flour, is iron deficient. Thirdly, excess calcium, fibre, antacid medication all block the uptake of iron; as does the lack of stomach acid.

Deficiency will lead to anaemia (lack of haemoglobin and oxygen carrying capacity of the blood) with consequent weakness and proneness to infection.

Women, because of the monthly loss of blood associated with the menstrual period, are more likely to suffer from anaemia than men. Other conditions, such as bleeding haemorrhoids, worm infestations, or other conditions causing blood loss, also contribute to anaemia.

Despite all this, the body does conserve iron very well, with a daily requirement of about 10 mg.

Excess of iron is less common, but exists where all cooking is done in iron vessels, or iron supplements are over-consumed. This accumulation of iron also occurs in people with deficiency in the iron transport mechanism leading to a condition called haemachromatosis, damaging the liver (cirrhosis), the pancreas (diabetes) and skin, causing a typical bronze discolouration.

Zinc

Like Magnesium, zinc is involved in the formation of numerous enzyme systems in the body, involving physical and mental functions.

- It is a necessary component of bone and tooth formation.
- It has antioxidant activity and forms part of the antioxidant enzyme, superoxide dismutase.
- In the developing fetus, zinc is involved in forming the skeleton, growth of the nervous system and assisting brain function.

Minerals
Zinc and Chromium

- It is necessary for cell growth, haemoglobin and production of hormones.
- It (not calcium) is responsible for the formation of strong nails, hair growth and integrity of the skin; all formed from a protein, keratin.
- It is involved in production and use of insulin.
- It is necessary for the senses of taste and smell.

Sources

The best sources of zinc are meat, eggs and sea foods; especially shellfish. Leafy green vegetables have less. There appears to be a widespread deficiency in the population, partly due to current farming practices with widespread use of artificial fertilisers. There is also widespread variation in the amount of zinc present in the soil. The other factor is the removal of what zinc there is in the food by processing methods.

The effect of deficiency is difficult to identify because zinc is involved in so many functions. Zinc status is best identified by laboratory testing of serum and intracellular zinc levels.

In men, the prostate gland has one of the highest concentrations of zinc in the body. It is responsible for the production of seminal fluid, in which the sperm swim and are nourished and is involved with the production of the male hormone, testosterone.

Zinc deficiency is associated with low sperm numbers and reduced sperm motility (ability of sperm to swim actively to reach and fertilise the female egg: the ovum).

Deficiency is also one of the many factors affecting potency, (male erectile power); hence the popularity of the oyster as an aphrodisiac, with its massive contribution of 50 mg of zinc in 100g (3½ ounces).

Let us not give all the credit to the oyster, when other shellfish can also offer substantial amounts of zinc.

[Not many years ago, most physicians wore pins behind the lapel of their jackets as instruments for testing nerve sensation. In these current days, of HIV and political correctness, the only use for the pins should be to extract a winkle from its shell.]

Toxicity of zinc is low. With a daily requirement of about 10 mg (more in people who are physically active), even doses of 500 mg appear to be non-toxic. Remember, however, that all these elements have an interplay and an excess of one can create imbalance of others; in the case of zinc, interference with the use of copper.

Chromium

Sources

This element is distributed widely in foods. Meat, fish – especially shellfish – are good sources, as are grains and vegetables.

- It is involved with the mechanism for maintaining blood glucose levels.
- Together with insulin, it is involved in the metabolism of glucose.
- It forms part of the Glucose Tolerance Factor.
- It is needed for normal blood lipid metabolism.
- It is essential for fatty acid metabolism and muscle growth.

Minerals
Chromium and Copper

Because of its wide distribution in food, deficiency of chromium should, like iron, be uncommon. Unfortunately, there are two factors which can cause severe deficiency. Firstly, although the body uses sugar (mainly glucose) as one of its fuels, it prefers to make it from the food we eat.

If we take in too much sugar in the diet, or foods, such as refined starches, which are rapidly turned into sugar, the control mechanism is overtaxed and chromium, of which we have little reserve, is rapidly used up. Secondly, all processed food is severely depleted of chromium. The result is a swinging of sugar levels from high to low, with consequent drop in energy. This causes the sufferer to seek some sugar-containing food "for energy" and so make matters worse. If this is continued, the tissues no longer retain the sensitivity to respond to insulin (insulin intolerance) and the condition of "age onset" diabetes develops. Chromium is established by laboratory measurement of serum levels. Daily requirement varies from 100-200mcg.

In the organic form in foods, chromium is non-toxic. In the supplement form of chromium polynicotinate, **(not picolinate of which there are some doubts about its safety)** even 1000mcg appears to be without ill-effect. It should be noted that other compounds of chromium, chromates, are not only highly toxic, but also carcinogenic.

Copper

- Copper is involved with the formation of red blood cells.
- It is a catalyst/moderator for the formation of water from hydrogen and oxygen at body temperature; (a reaction that would normally take place with explosive force!).
- It is involved in the use of iron for haemoglobin production.
- It is used in the formation of some brain neuro-transmitters, such as nor-adrenaline.
- Like iron, copper is moved to areas of damage (trauma) and is involved in producing enzymes concerned with cell respiration. Its requirement, therefore, is increased in athletes and during pregnancy and lactation.

Sources

Copper is most richly supplied by meat, offals and seafoods. It is present in small amounts in most vegetables and, nowadays, in households where the water supply comes through copper piping.

Copper is involved in so many different activities that deficiency is difficult to detect. The simplest test is measurement of copper in the blood serum.

Daily needs have been estimated as 2-3 mg; an amount that seems easily provided in the diet.

Copper in excess is toxic. Long ago, French wine growers used to spray grapes growing by the road side with copper sulphate, a mild poison, to prevent people from picking the grapes and eating them. Symptoms range from fatigue, irritability, depression, lack of concentration to gastrointestinal upset and damage to the liver. An uncommon

Minerals

Manganese and Iodine

familial inherited disorder known as Wilson's disease, results from progressive accumulation of copper in the tissues including the red blood cells, kidney, liver and brain. Another condition, Indian childhood cirrhosis, occurring in Asian communities, is of similar nature.

Manganese

- Manganese is essential for fat synthesis and for the conversion of simple essential fatty acids to more complex forms necessary for all hormone production and for the fats in breast milk.
- Manganese takes part in the synthesis of structural cell proteins.
- It is involved with glycogen storage in the liver and for normal glucose metabolism.
- It takes part in the formation and toughness of bone (without manganese bone would be very brittle) and in the formation of joint cartilage.
- It is a co-factor in numerous enzymes involved in growth and is part, as is zinc, of the antioxidant enzyme, super oxide dismutase (SOD).
- It is involved in the function of the nervous system and energy production.
- It activates enzymes enabling the use of vitamins B, Biotin, choline and vitamin C.

Sources

Manganese is obtained from all leafy green vegetables, whole grains and tea. Soil deficiencies can influence availability.

Deficiency is difficult to identify because of its multi-factorial function. The daily requirement is estimated to be between 2-5 mg, and higher in athletes.

Toxicity of manganese is considered to be very low by the oral route, although large supplements can interfere with iron absorption. Inhalation of manganese dust, as has happened in the steel and chemical industries, has been known to cause insanity.

Iodine

Iodine is essential for the formation of the group of hormones manufactured by the thyroid gland. The function is to control the rate of metabolism (the sum total of chemical activity in the body) of all the cells.

Sources

The best sources are all kinds of seafood, both fish of all kinds and maritime plants. Even living by the sea and breathing the sea air will provide enough iodine for our needs. Soil content varies and in many parts of the world, including the central parts of England, the European Alps, the Himalayas, some central parts of North and South America, parts of new Zealand, can be totally lacking.

When there is a shortage of iodine the thyroid gland, in an effort to supply sufficient hormone, will enlarge. This shows as a visible swelling on the front of the neck; goitre. Years ago, in a part of central England lacking in iodine, this condition was described as Derbyshire Neck. The effect of deficiency in the infant is cretinism, with retardation of physical and mental development. In the adult, the condition is myxoedema. The individual is slow, physically and mentally, cold with a slow pulse. The skin in myxoedema is typically

Minerals
Iodine, Molybdenum and Boron

puffy due to an accumulation of a form of gel under the skin. Both conditions can be cured (if cretinism is detected sufficiently early) by the administration of iodine. The addition of a small amount of iodine to table salt (iodised salt) has made a huge contribution to the reduction of these conditions (particularly goitre).

Nowadays, most cases of adult myxoedema result from an auto-immune disorder of the thyroid gland – thyroiditis – and not iodine deficiency.

Daily needs are quite small, in the region of 150mcg or less and is easily obtained in a diet containing foods of maritime origin.

Toxicity of iodine is low up to a daily intake of 1,000mcg (2,000mcg in athletes who lose much in sweat). Above that, there is a likelihood of damage to the thyroid gland, with resultant *diminution* of hormone production.

Molybdenum

This element forms part of three essential protective enzymes. It is also one of the components maintaining the health of the mucous membranes throughout the body.

Sources

Molybdenum is found in many foods including whole grains and pulses.

Effects of deficiency have not been described but have been observed in some cases of excess mucous production, whether in the sinuses, lungs, digestive tract or genito-urinary tract.

The daily requirements are not known for certain; probably about 150mcg.

Toxicity of molybdenum is very low but high doses, in excess of 10 mg, can cause arthritic pain. In reindeer, excess has been shown to displace chromium and to induce type II diabetes.

Boron

This element is connected with the manufacture of hormones, particularly involving the use of calcium, phosphorus and manganese in bone formation; also for muscle development. Boron is also involved in the production of other steroid hormones; notably testosterone and a form of oestrogen (oestradiol).

The study of this element dates back only 20 years. As a result specific deficiency has not been properly identified, but because of its involvement with the use of calcium, phosphorus and manganese, may well be implicated with the development of osteoporosis, as well as some forms of arthritis and raised blood pressure.

Sources

Sources of boron lie in most foods, but are richest in nuts, dried fruits and pulses, as well as leafy vegetables and fresh fruits.

The daily requirement is estimated to be about 2mg.

Toxicity is low, but high doses (50 mg or more) are thought to interfere with the effects of some of the B-complex vitamins.

Cobalt

This is the element around which the molecule of vitamin B_{12} is built.

Minerals
Boron, Cobalt and Selenium

It seems to be present in all foods. Deficiency is considered to be unlikely, in view of the minute amount required, (less than half of 1 millionth of a gram).

Selenium

Highly toxic in quantity, selenium in trace amounts is essential to health, having a multitude of functions. It is to be found in every cell in the body; most abundantly in hair, kidneys and testes.

Together with vitamin E, it is involved in the production of Co-enzyme Q10 (CoQ10) and glutathione peroxidaze (GSH-Px). These are enzymes acting as antioxidants, with additional requirement of vitamins A and C, to control activity of necessary but potentially dangerous free radicals.

Selenium is required for prostaglandin production and ensuring hormone balance. This includes the production of healthy sperm (and, therefore, fertility) in men as well as trouble-free menstruation and, subsequently, menopause in women.

With another enzyme, glutathione s-transferase (GST), selenium acts to detoxify and eliminate toxic chemicals, including the heavy metals: lead, mercury and cadmium and to protect against radiation.

Selenium is important for a healthy heart and for the health of eyes, skin and hair.

Selenium, together with vitamin E, protects against infection. It is involved with the mechanism affecting the different kinds of protective white cells in the blood and, therefore, its role in protecting against cancer.

Selenium is involved in the synthesis of proteins and other biochemical compounds.

Selenium is absolutely vital for energy production. Without it the circulating thyroid hormone would not be activated by the energy components in the cells (mitochondria). The result, if not death, would be gross physical and mental debility.

Availability of selenium varies greatly. It seems that over thousands of years, soils have become depleted and, as in the case of iodine, may in some areas be totally lacking. The present day fashion of 'refining' foods has made the situation worse. All vegetables should contain selenium, but not requiring the element for themselves, can thrive on selenium deficient soils.

Sources

Because the seas contain selenium, the most reliable sources are fish of all kinds, including shellfish and maritime plants such as samphire, various seaweeds and algae.

Deficiency in selenium can be associated with low energy, increased susceptibility to infections, risk of cancer, premature ageing and, in men, reduced fertility.

The daily requirement is estimated to be between 60 - 80 mcg.

What do we need to eat to give us our daily selenium requirement?

Minerals

Selenium and Vanadium

2 free range eggs (or 20 of the other kind)

or

3 oysters

or

2 large scallops

or

4 brazil nuts

or

8 walnuts

Because vegetables vary according to soil and type of manuring one cannot specify type or weight – but insist on variety – preferably organically grown.

Vanadium

This metal has long been regarded by veterinarians as being essential for animal health, affecting reproduction, bone and tooth formation and development of feathers and fur. Some bacteria use it and the blood of the sea-squirt – a degenerate survivor of the ancestors of vertebrates – is green because the oxygen carrying pigment is formed around vanadium, unlike the more efficient iron-based red-coloured haemoglobin in ourselves and many other creatures.

Only fairly recently, has research shown that vanadium is also a essential element in human nutrition.

The total amount in the body is very small, probably 25 grams (less than one ounce), but is widely distributed with concentrations in bone and fat.

Information gathered so far indicates that vanadium is involved in fat metabolism, the production of red blood cells, growth and reproduction. It is also involved with calcium in the mechanisms for controlling blood sugar and cholesterol levels, protecting against insulin resistance.

Sources

As with selenium, availability of vanadium varies greatly according to soil content. It is present in all plants in small and differing amounts, according to species, but is more available in fats and vegetable oils, especially unsaturated oils, olive oil and nuts; also in oily fish and shellfish.

Deficiency of vanadium has not been properly identified but it is thought that it may be associated with raised levels of blood sugar and cholesterol and (by inference) increased risk of heart disease.

Toxicity of vanadium in humans has not yet been demonstrated, although some forms of mental illness, depression and bipolar disorder (manic depression) have been linked to raised levels in the blood.

The daily requirement is not yet known, but the 2mg present in the average diet is, in the light of present knowledge, presumed to be adequate.

Minerals
Fluoride, Arsenic, Silicon, Bromine (Bromide)

Fluoride (Fluorine)

Like chloride, fluoride is an *anion*, electrically negatively charged. It is essential for the formation of strong bones and healthy teeth.

Availability varies in different soils and in different parts of the world. In many countries, it is added to the water supply, as sodium fluoride, as an aid to prevent tooth decay. The actual daily need seems not to be known, but why not surmise? Sea water, from which all life originated currently contains fluorine in a concentration of 1.3 parts per million. A water supply with a level below this (perhaps $1/3$) would seem to be reasonable.

Fluoride in excess is toxic. It first shows as pitting and brown-staining of developing teeth. Gross excess, as evidenced among the El Molo people in Kenya causes softening of the bones, especially of the legs, with characteristic bowing. Examination of skeletons of people found in prehistoric graves in Bahrein revealed gross arthritis of the joints and fusion of the spinal vertebrae. This was the result of their drinking water from wells with a high fluoride content.

Arsenic

Usually regarded, correctly, as a poison. Arsenic is now considered essential for growth. It is widely distributed in soils and is present in minute quantities in vegetables. The daily requirement is, at present, unknown.

Silicon

After oxygen, silicon is the most commonly occurring element on the planet. It exists in many different forms: in rocks, sand, quartz, opals, clays and volcanic and diatomaceous earths such as zeolites and bentonite.

In humans, in the form of silicon dioxide (silica, silicic acid) SiO_2, it is present in minute amounts in skin, lungs and extracellular (ouside the cells) matrix and, until recently, has been considered to be non essential, having no observed biological activity. Recent research, on the contrary, reveals that silicon exerts a powerful influence on all tissues, behaving on the one hand like an antioxidant to prevent tissue damage and on the other hand as a chelator to remove heavy metals and other toxic substances from the body.

Sources

Silicon occurs in all plants in varying amounts (the "hairs" on leaves of such plants as the stinging nettle, Urtica urens and comfrey, Symphytum, consists of hollow needles of amost pure silica). All meats and fish also provide silicon in smaller amounts.

Daily requirements are, as yet, unknown. Deficiency when eating correctly is unlikely because of the ubiquitous nature of the element, but constant reliance on refined foods obviously presents a danger.

Like all elements, essential or otherwise, when inhaled in the gaseous state or as finely divided dust, silica can lodge in the lungs. There it destroys the elastic tissue, producing a condition of fibrosis; the silicosis of miners.

Bromine (Bromide)

Like chloride and fluoride, it is an *anion* and, therefore, electrically active. It appears in very small amounts in maritime foods and appears not to be biologically active at that level.

In larger amounts, such as medication with bromide preparations, it can displace iodine and interfere with thyroid function.

In the gaseous form it is extremely toxic and corrosive.

Strontium

This element is widely distributed in small amounts. It can displace calcium and is to be found wherever calcium is present, but does not pose a problem.

Toxicity is assumed to be low (except in the radioactive form).

A Miscellany

Tin, germanium and nickel have been shown to be important for animal growth. The effects in humans have yet to be established.

Chapter 9

The Toxic Metals

The Toxic Metals (The Heavy Metals)
Lead

All the elements essential to all living creatures, including ourselves, exist almost uniformly in the sea. They are less evenly distributed on land; some, scarce and in pockets, have only appeared in the environment in the past 4-5,000 years since Man has begun to extract these metals and to spread them around the earth. They include aluminium, barium, bismuth, gold and silver, which are considered to have relatively low toxicity; others, including antimony, cadmium, lead, mercury, tellurium and tin are poisonous; both life-threatening and life-shortening.

Interestingly, elements in mammalian blood (not that of 'western' man) are present in the same proportions that probably prevailed in the seas of the Cambrian Era (500,000,000 years ago) which are estimated to have been about one third as salty as today's seas.

Today, we have more toxic elements in our systems than did our ancestors. Although we have mechanisms for eliminating toxic trace metals through the sweat, kidneys, bile and digestive tract, the levels in the environment have increased.

Lead

This metal has no known biological benefit. It is poisonous to all tissues, but lodges preferentially in bone and brain. Lead was probably a major cause of the fall of Ancient Rome; with the advent of water supplied through lead piping, wine stored and served in leaden vessels, the build up of this toxic metal led to weakness and dementia.

In England, cider, a drink made from apples, has always been more popular in the countryside than in the towns. Until the end of the nineteenth century, the juice from the pressed apples would run from the press down runnels made of wood and lined with lead to the barrels where it would be fermented. Because the apple juice is acidic, some of the lead would inevitably be dissolved. The consumption of cider, which is a very effective thirst-quencher, was very high among the hard working country men. It is probably a contributory factor to the town dwellers' view of the country 'bumpkin' (stupid fellow).

Recent evidence indicates that lead, accumulated in the womb of an already contaminated mother, is a likely factor in the children's developing schizophrenia in later life.

Hazards in the United Kingdom used to include the emissions of motor vehicles using leaded petrol – thankfully, now reducing; not only inhaled, but by children in poor areas playing in the streets who would pick up the contaminated dirt on their hands and (inevitably) convey it to their mouths. Leaded housepaint in older houses was another danger (as is its removal nowadays, requiring great care). Another source of lead poisoning is found in older houses in soft-water areas, such as Glasgow in Scotland, where the water is supplied through lead piping. The acidity of the water is sufficient to dissolve a small amount of lead into the water, causing a gradual accumulation in the body. Happily, these faults are gradually being eliminated to the benefit of future generations.

The Toxic Metals (The Heavy Metals)
Cadmium and Mercury

Cadmium

This element appears to have no biological value. It has proved to be a major hazard in cadmium-using industries such as electroplating and battery and plastic manufacture. This is associated with diseases of the kidney, prostate and lung. Smokers are at risk, because tobacco is a source of cadmium. This heavy metal lodges in the lung, where it causes local irritation and, in the susceptible individual, destroys the elastic tissue of the lung with the development of emphysema; in others, lung cancer. It is a factor in the development of hypertension (high blood pressure).

Recent studies[1] on female rats have shown that cadmium even in minute amounts behaves like oestrogen, promoting earlier puberty, denser mammary tissue and heavier wombs.

This effect has not yet been observed in humans, but is a matter for concern as plants take up cadmium from phosphate fertilisers.

There is, however, evidence that supports the inference that cadmium increases the risk of oestrogen-related cancers. A study conducted in British Columbia[2] of over two thousand women, revealed that those who had begun smoking within five years of the first menstrual period were 70% more likely to develop breast cancer than those who had never smoked.

Mercury

This, the third heavy metal, also has no biological value. The effects were first noticed in industry and chemical works. Mercury fumes can be inhaled and the metal can be transmitted though the skin. Some small amounts occur in food but can be excreted. Mercury, when absorbed, leaves the blood rapidly and locates itself into muscle and brain. In the muscles, it produces progressive weakness and inco-ordination; in the brain, can lead to insanity – the Mad Hatter's disease of old time top-hat makers who formed the animal fur into felt by rubbing in mercury with their hands.

The source that affects most individuals today is from metallic tooth fillings; an amalgam comprised principally of mercury and silver. For the most part, these fillings (which have been used for the greater part of a century) remain inert. Occasionally, they corrode and mercury is released, with sometimes disastrous results.

Mercury in the organic form, ethyl mercury (thiomersal, UK – thimerosal, US), is present in many vaccines as a preservative. It is still widely used, particularly in the UK, despite concerns regarding the safety of these vaccines (the developing brain of the infant is especially vulnerable) and of the fact that they have been withdrawn from use in most of the developed countries[3].

---

[1] *New Scientist, July 2003*

[2] *Lancet, October 2002*

[3] *Belatedly, new legislation in the UK has prohibited the continued use of mercury preservatives in vaccines. September 2004.*

The Toxic Metals (The Heavy Metals)
Aluminium and Beryllium

Aluminium

Why this element is lumped together with the "heavy" metals, I don't know. What I do know however is that it is toxic, but in a sneakier fashion than the preceding culprits.

Although there is a little in the food we eat (aluminium is very widely distributed in the soils of this world) the principle source of contamination comes from aluminium cooking vessels (including coated "non-stick" types) and aluminium foil used for wrapping food prior to cooking. Deodorant preparations contain aluminium salts and in some susceptible people, aluminium is absorbed through the skin.

I said that the effects were sneakier, in that they are not so clear-cut. In a small child, the appetite is often reduced and the child takes an abnormally long time to eat even a small amount. Itchiness of the skin, particularly around the eyes and nose is often present. In the adult, digestive symptoms are prominent, ranging from diminished appetite, a feeling of food's forming a lump and sticking behind the sternum (breast-bone), belching, acidity and heart burn, colic, erratic bowel function and constipation. In addition to all: lack of energy.

Removing aluminium from the kitchen produces a rapid response in susceptible children. Adults are slower but do show a definite improvement to the change.

Beryllium

This very light metal, which is highly toxic, has only become an increasing hazard within the last fifty years or so. It is used as a moderator in nuclear reactors and the oxide is used in industry as a hardener for special steels. Nowadays it extends into the lives of all of us, being used in the phosphor coatings in fluorescent lighting and television tubes.

Inhalation of dust or fumes of beryllium salts causes a disease of the lungs, berylliosis, in which granulomata[1] are formed in the lungs. Cuts from beryllium coated glass (e.g. broken fluorescent tubes) cause similar lesions on the skin which are difficult to eradicate – a strong argument for the careful disposal of spent fluorescent tubes; never to be broken up and used in landfills, as seems to be current practice.

> **All the toxic elements tend to accumulate and to lodge in the system. Elimination is very slow, although improved where the level of nutrition is good and the individual is physically active. Fortunately, there are methods of chemical combination (chelation) which render these elements soluble and, therefore, removable. Such chelation therapy requires very expert supervision if only to prevent removal of all the beneficial and necessary minerals at the same time.**

---

[1] *granuloma: a pathological term referring to a localised collection of granulation tissue (rough, lumpy) caused by infection or by invasion by a foreign body.*

Chapter 10

Exercise

Exercise

The body rusts away quicker than it wears away.

For a healthy existence, we need three things: good nutrition, adequate sleep and regular, moderate exercise.

During the millions of years of evolution, Man was forced to be physically active: in his quest for food, whether foraging or hunting, building shelter and, in his turn, often fleeing from other predators bigger and fiercer than himself.

Nowadays, we have machines to work for us. To make a journey we do not have to walk. There are motor cars, buses, trains and aircraft. In the home, we have washing machines, dishwashers and vacuum cleaners. Heating the house is done at the turn of a switch, so that we no longer have to fetch and carry fuel or to stoke the fires. In these conditions, our bodies do not even have to generate extra heat to combat low external temperatures. Lifts and escalators can help us to avoid the physical effort of climbing stairs.

This resultant physical inactivity is costing us dearly.

Incidentally, for exercise read physical activity. It need not be associated with working in a gymnasium but rather with any pursuit that one can enjoy.

For instance, a brisk walk of 20-30 minutes daily, swimming, playing tennis or golf a couple of times in a week, horse-riding, even mowing the lawn, all constitute exercise.

Cardiovascular illness.

Apart from what has been said about the relationship between poor nutrition and cardiovascular disease, it is known that lack of exercise is also a contributor. Conversely, appropriate regular, moderate exercise is beneficial in reducing the incidence of heart attacks and increasing life expectancy.

The heart after all is a muscular pump. Like all muscles, it responds to extra demand made on it to develop strength and stamina.

Circulation of blood to the extremities is augmented by the muscles of arms and legs which act as auxiliary pumps and assist the work of the heart by improving the circulation to more remote parts.

The lymphatic circulation in particular is dependent on muscular effort. Lymph is a colourless liquid which seeps from the blood through the capillary walls to bathe the tissues bringing oxygen and nutrients and removing waste products, finally returning to re-enter the blood-stream via a large vein near the heart. Because the lymphatic system has no pump of its own, circulation of this life-maintaining fluid can only be effectively maintained by muscular activity.

Bone demineralization (osteoporosis) and fractures.

Think of the bones as levers and the muscles as motors. If the motor is powerful and the lever is fragile, strong effort will break it. Fortunately, bone is "plastic" and is capable of responding to heavier

Exercise
Bone Demineralisation (Osteoporosis), Arthritis and mental function

demands made on it by increasing its size, density and therefore, strength.

Conversely, lack of use, lack of muscular exercise, results in loss of bone density.

A few years ago in London, excavation was taking place at a site of a new building. In the process, an old cemetery was uncovered dating back some two hundred years. Anthropologists flocking to the site were amazed to note that the bones of the women of the time were much thicker and stronger than those of comparative age living today. It is most unlikely that the women of the earlier time enjoyed more adequate diet than what is presently available. Their comparative lack of height indicates that. No, the difference in bone density reflects the much greater physical effort enforced by the life-style of that time.

Current advice on prevention of osteoporosis by increasing intake of calcium by consumption of milk and milk products is wrong. Calcium is only one of many minerals involved in bone formation (see the section on minerals and their functions) and excess of calcium can cause demineralisation of bone. A report in 1997 on the "Nurses Health Study" involving some 100,000 nurses over 20 years and continuing, shows that post-menopausal women who take 2 glasses (approximately 16oz/600ml) or more, perhaps added to tea or coffee[1], are 40% *more likely* to suffer hip fractures than those who take none.

---

[1] *This could include "altered" milk, i.e. cheese, yoghurt etc.*

Arthritis and joint disease.

Whereas moderate regular physical activity stimulates repair and maintenance of joint surfaces, with production of the lubricating (synovial) fluid, constant overload will cause excessive wear and tear and development of osteo-arthritis. This effect is enhanced by poor diet. Antioxidants and other protective substances found in leafy green vegetables as well as the essential fatty acids (notably the omega 3 group from marine sources) play a vital role, helping also to preserve the suppleness of soft tissues, joints and tendons.

Rheumatoid arthritis is a different condition. It is an auto immune response, where the body reacts against itself. The origin is unknown but may be initiated by multiple factors, including allergy and certain types of bacterial, viral or even fungal infections. Clinical experience shows that adopting a healthy diet approaching that of our early ancestors can produce some improvement. My own opinion is that eating healthily from an early age would be an effective preventive to this crippling disorder that affects about 1% of the population with a bias of 2:1 towards women.

Exercise and mental function.

I often think that muscles, when active, behave like glands inducing improved functioning elsewhere.

Many patients of mine, high-ranking business people whose time is so precious that they would not give you five minutes unless you paid for it, nevertheless will take a whole hour out of a busy

Exercise
Stimulates mental ability

day in order to exercise. To gain the body beautiful? Not at all, but because it sharpens them mentally. They can think more clearly and effectively.

> **Although, in the UK, physical education and games periods are incorporated in the school syllabus, there has been an increasing tendency, by many schools, to "steal" these (as well as times for religious instruction) for academic work. The effect has been to produce the opposite of what was intended, by a lowering of intellectual ability and attention and increasing boredom and difficult behaviour. This has imposed a heavier burden on teachers, trying for ever to reach higher standards, and stress on the pupils, whose response is greatly increased truancy.**

In those schools where games are encouraged and physical education maintained, not only are the children fitter, more physically co-ordinated and alert, but calmer, happier and more capable, with less time allocated, of *greater* academic achievement; all with less pressure on the pupil to "succeed".

Where physical activity in school is encouraged, it tends to be maintained after school hours. Children play more and remain physically active. Conversely, where physical activity in school is low, so after-school activity, especially in the group of 15 plus years, is diminished, being replaced with time spent on sedentary television watching or computer fixation.

No wonder that, in Britain, one child in three is overweight, developing an increasing amount of antisocial behaviour, depression and, of course, the threat of future ill-health.

Exercise for most people is mood enhancing.

Without it they feel unwell and become depressed, indicating that not all forms of depression are psychological in origin or a reaction to circumstances, but a chemical state.

For all of us, some form of exercise is necessary for good health and a sense of well-being.

For any one of you engaged in vigorous activities – all forms of athletics or undergoing physical training (hopefully, with expert guidance), here is some important information:

- **Excessive or inappropriate exercise is harmful.**

In 1948, before suitable protection was available, there was in Britain, an epidemic of polio-myelitis; quite frighteningly savage in its effect. The big surprise was that the people most vulnerable were professional athletes and other sporting types. These were more likely to be affected by paresis (permanent weakness) and paralysis than their more sedentary contemporaries. It should not have been so, but in those days, less was known than today about the science of exercise. Those individuals who had been overtraining and were without correct nutritional support suffered as a result.

Lesson: Never train in ignorance.

Always seek a competent teacher.

Exercise
Seek competent advice

- Because heavy exercise increases water loss from the skin through sweating and also from the lungs, drink at least 280ml (half a pint) of water, not immediately, *but half an hour before exercising.* This allows time for the liquid to pass through the stomach into the small intestine, where it is absorbed and passed into the system. Follow this after exercise by having another drink to replenish the fluids that have been lost.

- Do not take salt, sodium chloride, to replace that lost in sweat. Most of us have a more than adequate intake of salt and the body is very efficient at conserving sodium (see the section on minerals). Water is your only need. Equally, avoid swamping your system with much publicised, often very expensive, patent mineral mixtures without seeking professional advice; preferably with some laboratory evidence of what may be your personal needs.

- Try to make it possible to *rest immediately* after heavy and/or sustained activity. This is most important advice which is seldom offered even by professional trainers. A relatively short period of between 20 and 30 minutes will suffice.

During any kind of sustained activity, muscle tissue is broken down and waste products are created. These substances, if allowed to accumulate, cause the aching and stiffness often experienced some hours (and sometimes days) later. Interestingly, it is the presence of these same substances that stimulates the repair of damaged muscle tissue and encourages the growth of new blood vessels and so increase the blood supply.

Here is the catch. This can only occur efficiently during periods of rest or sleep, when new muscle fibres begin to grow and new blood vessels are formed to bring in greater supplies of nutrients and to remove more efficiently, any waste products. If rest is omitted, the prolonged presence of waste products causes inflammation and the formation of scar tissue – nature's emergency repair material. The effect is to produce bulk, giving the impression of increased muscle size, but no increase in muscle power. The result is a loss of suppleness; the sort of stiffening often described as "muscle bound".

- The current fashion of "stoking-up" before any activity with very large intakes of carbohydrates, starch in some form, can be wrong and even detrimental to health and performance. It is true that the carbohydrate reserve in muscle, glycogen, is converted to glucose and used by the muscles during periods of *very high* physical effort. This fuel would become unavailable after about two hours of such exertion. Thereafter, effort can only be sustained at a lower level by the body's main fuel – fat.

Mind over matter

Is fatigue all in the mind? It sets in before the muscle nutrients are expended – some 30-50% being held in reserve – and before toxins resulting from muscular effort have risen to dangerous levels. I am convinced that this is a safety mechanism, part of a "Survival Kit" inherited from our early ancestors and designed to provide sufficient reserves of energy to get us out of trouble in an emergency. Imagine the hunter wending his weary way home

Exercise
Mind over matter

who is suddenly attacked by a predator, animal or human and who is immediately able to summon the necessary strength to fight or flee. This mechanism is under the control of the central nervous system. It explains how some modern athletes can, by sheer will power, at the end of a gruelling race when all are flagging, overcome their own feeling of exhaustion and produce that extra burst of power that enables them to win.

However much time and effort we spend on developing a healthy musculature, it is the **Mind** that dictates the strength we can exert and for how long. I learned that when farming. Men slighter than I (and I am no Hercules) were lifting weights of one hundred weight (50kg) and more, which I *thought* I could not; until I thought to myself "if they can, I can" and did.

I remember an incident reported in a newspaper some years ago. A child had been run over and trapped under the wheel of a motor car. The mother, a slightly-built lady of about five feet two inches (1m57.5) in height grasped the front bumper bar of the car, lifted it and rolled the car off her child. Later, it was discovered that the intense force exerted had caused several crush fractures of the mother's spine: a true example of Mind over Matter.

- Truly, proper muscular development and use, combined with correct nutrition, will lead to an enhanced state of physical and mental health. The truism *mens sana in corpore sano* – a healthy mind in a healthy body – was supposedly composed in the first century AD by a Roman satirist, Juvenal (which, I suspect, that he derived from an earlier Greek philosopher – plagiarism is not a new invention).

Conditions stemming from unhealthy eating include diabetes, raised blood-pressure and high cholesterol levels. All of these can be helped by appropriate exercise so that raised blood sugar is lowered as is cholesterol and resting blood pressure. These effects are immediate as can be shown by testing before and after an exercise session. It goes without saying, however, that for permanent improvement it is important to implement the pattern of healthy nutrition, previously described.

Obesity, the curse of our present society and beginning to become a world-wide problem is primarily the effect of incorrect diet. Exercise alone is ineffective to produce loss of weight and, unsupervised, even dangerous, but it is, however, of real benefit when combined with healthy nutrition.

Chapter 11

Nutrition for the Family

Nutrition for the Family
The parents

Before pregnancy

In the majority of cases, marriage results in procreation – and so a new human being is born.

Quite properly, consideration has always been given to the health of the woman, both before and especially during pregnancy. The importance of the health of the father has, so far, been totally ignored.

Think of it. Each is contributing, in equal amounts, material to form a new human being. True, the egg (ovum) from the woman is massive – at least a hundred times larger – compared with the sperm cell from the man, but the size of the nucleus of each containing all the important genetic material is similar in both. The difference in size is largely due to the fact that the ovum contains organs called mitochondria – almost, but not quite absent in the sperm. They are derived almost entirely from the mother and are the energy producing structures within the cell. The rest of the difference in size results from the presence of a very large fuel reserve (rather like the yolk in the egg of a chicken) which provides the initial energy for growth before the developing embryo can attach itself to the mother.

For a fit and healthy child to be conceived, it is essential that both prospective parents should also be fit and healthy.[1]

Question: If I want to have children, what should be done?
Answer: Ideally, you should both work to improve your diet for at least 3–4 months before conception.

At the same time, each of you should visit your general physician for an overall physical check, including laboratory measurement of mineral, vitamin and essential fatty acid levels[2]; then, if necessary and under professional guidance, taking whatever supplementation may be indicated.

> I strongly recommend all parents and prospective parents to obtain and read Brain Child by Tony Buzan. It is an absolute necessity (and an ideal wedding present!) – see bibliography.

This may seem to be a overly fussy approach to what is a natural event. The truth is that even among couples with no known fertility problems, there is only a 25% chance of pregnancy each month (although in the end they may succeed).

More importantly, many instances of miscarriage have been laid at the door of malnutrition and a corresponding deficiency in the cell donated by either parent. Indeed, it is considered among doctors that very many miscarriages occur without being noticed; just thought to be a 'missed period'.

Down's syndrome used to be thought to result from some fault in the mother as she aged. Certainly, where a woman who has had children previously and, because of inadequate diet, becomes physically depleted, this may be the case. On the other hand, there are countless examples of women who, in their late 40s and early 50s, have borne healthy offspring. It is now recognised that many cases of Down's syndrome are the result of a fault in the father.

---

[1] Foresight – see bibliography

[2] Unfortunately, this facility is not at present available in Britain on the National Health Service. A situation, that for the good of everyone will, hopefully, be corrected.

Nutrition for the Family
The mother and baby

Spina bifida is a developmental fault in which the spinal cord and coverings fail to form properly. It can often result in severe handicap and, sometimes, premature death. It is now known to be caused by dietary deficiency; principally, but not solely a lack of folic acid, one of the B vitamins. A much more serious deformity, having the same cause is anencephaly, where the brain fails to develop and the infant cannot survive.

A joint study from New York University, Columbia University's College of Physicians and Surgeons and Israel's Ministry of Health has found that children fathered by men older than 50 were three times as likely to suffer from schizophrenia than those children whose fathers were aged 25 or less. This would again appear to implicate a deterioration in the nutritional state of the father with increasing age.

During pregnancy

The nutritional requirements of the pregnant mother will not rise appreciably for the first 3–4 months and, provided that she is eating correctly in the first place, should not alter her nutritional intake.

If you are eating properly, you shouldn't "eat for two" – you will only increase your chances of putting on unnecessary extra weight. Increase the amount you eat after 4 months, because your energy and nutrient needs will rise rapidly as the developing fetus will be growing fast, as will the uterus (womb) and the placenta. It is during the last

---

Two points to ponder:

1 Hyperemesis Gravidarum – vomiting of pregnancy

Nausea and vomiting occur so frequently in the early weeks of pregnancy as to be considered normal. Is it, as some authorities argue, the mother's initial reaction to the presence of a foreign body before adjusting to its presence? I am not sure.

2 Cravings of pregnancy

Cravings are not inevitable, but not uncommon. They can sometimes be quite bizarre, such as a desire to eat chalk or drink vinegar. More commonly simply to over indulge in every day foods. Are they triggered subconsciously by a nutritional deficiency (precipitated by the increased anabolic[1] demand) which the body is trying, in an unfocussed way to correct? I think so.

---
[1] *anabolic: building up of complex substances in living matter.*

---

5 months that the growing baby will increase in size from approximately 0.5 kg (1lb) to 3.4-4kg (7 1/2-9lb). There is also an increase in the size of the uterus, now a large muscular bag weighing approximately 1 kg (2 lb) containing 1.5 litres of amniotic fluid weighing 1.5 kg (3.3lb), plus the placenta weighing 500g (1 lb). Added to this should be an accumulation of special fats in the breasts and under the skin, which are intended to supply

the essential fatty acids in the milk for nourishing the baby; providing the materials for continuing development of brain and nerve tissue, as well as fuel for energy for growth in the whole organism.

This means that at the time the baby is due to arrive, the mother will be at least 11-13.5kg (25-30lb) above her normal weight. Much of this extra weight would be lost at the birth itself, with a subsequent further loss over the next few weeks as the uterus is reabsorbed and restored to its normal size.

After the baby is born the mother's energy and nutritional requirements will still be moderately raised because of her need to produce milk for the growing baby's needs, (a breast fed baby will double its weight at approximately six months). Lactation requires considerable energy, 1000 Kcal per day or more. This and the fact that the mother's metabolism is working at a higher level, restores her more rapidly to her normal pre-pregnancy weight and configuration.

The Baby

The size of the baby at birth is important[1]. In a healthy, well nourished mother, the rate of growth of the fetus is rapid; reaching an ideal birth weight of 3.4-4kg (7 1/2-9lb).

These people who were well-nourished in the womb and after birth have, in later life, greater resilience to poor living conditions. They remain healthier and are at a lower risk of coronary heart disease than those who grew more slowly in the womb, with a consequent lighter birth weight. Of the latter, those who made a rapid weight gain between the ages of 1-12 years are the most susceptible to subsequent development of coronary heart disease, obesity and diabetes.

The size of the baby at birth is not influenced by the size of the father, but by the size of the mother, as well as by her nutritional state. In other words, a woman whose height of 5 feet (1m 52) has been determined by her genes, not malnutrition, would give birth to a smaller, lighter baby than a woman of 6 feet (1m 83).

Think about it. It makes good sense. Horse breeders and others concerned with livestock have long known this. For instance, a small pony mare mated to a large shire stallion, will give birth to a foal of a size appropriate to her own; in other words, the same as if the sire had been pony size. If this were not so, the result would be disastrous; not to say uncomfortable!

Lactation

Human milk is designed specifically for the human infant:

1 To supply nutritional needs;
2 To aid proper development and population of the bacterial content (flora) of the digestive tract ensuring correct digestive function, while inhibiting development of disease-producing (pathogenic) bacteria;

---

[1] "Figures from the World Health Organisation show that in 1992 the UK had the highest rate of low birth weight babies in the European Union; the UK's rate was on a par with Albania"
Growing up in Britain a book by the British Medical Association, 1999

Nutrition for the Family
Mother and baby – Lactation

3 To provide protection of the infant while its own, initially undeveloped, immune system can be evolved.

All mammals rely on bacteria in the digestive tract for assistance in the digestion of food and for the production of protective substances, e.g. vitamin K.

The milk delivered in the first few days to the infant, the colostrum, is very special[1]. Although small in amount, compared to the quantities of milk produced later, it contains relatively large amounts of retinol (vitamin A)[2] carotenes and vitamins; all antioxidants with protective qualities. Colostrum is also rich in antibodies from the mother, providing protection from various infections.

As lactation proceeds, the quantity of milk increases and the content of individual constituents changes. For instance, the levels of vitamin A and the carotenes gradually fall, while the calcium rises as does the fat content (and so, the energy content and supply of the structural fatty acids for brain and body growth). These changes continue throughout lactation, adjusting the formulation to meet the differing requirements at each stage of growth. The new-born baby has little or no enzyme for digesting fat (lipase). This is generously supplied in the breast milk and ensures that the fats in the milk are very efficiently digested and absorbed.

A natural analogy to the changes in composition of breast milk with time would be the way that certain birds (tits) feed their chicks with different insects at different times: spiders for some days, followed by caterpillars, then by flying insects. There seems to be a pattern to this (I am sure your local friendly bird-watcher or ornithologist would be pleased to explain) which meets the needs of the developing chicks at different stages of growth[3].

Milk sugar (lactose) is much higher in breast than in cows' milk and is important for the growth of bifido bacteria in the large intestine with the production of acids which suppress the growth of pathogenic bacteria.

Iron in breast milk is low, which is a factor in suppressing growth of pathogenic bacteria and certain yeasts (such as Candida) but a substance, lactoferrin, assures sufficient absorption of the low levels of iron present without risk.

Another valuable component of breast milk is a host of white blood cells derived from the mother. They are very numerous in colostrum and have the ability to gobble up pathogenic bacteria, such as E. coli and yeasts such as Candida albicans. (As these living cells stick to glass, expressed breast milk should be contained in plastic and used soon after; they are killed by heating and freezing.)

---

[1] Veterinary surgeons are well aware that when a foal or calf is born, if it does not receive the colostrum from its mother it will fail to thrive or even die soon after birth.
[2] Proliferation and migration of the cells of nerves and brain require vitamin A. It is needed for the growth and development of the cardio vascular system, as well as the development of the pancreas and those cells that produce insulin. See the section on vitamins for more information on the many functions of vitamin A.

[3] I am indebted to my son Peter for this information.

Nutrition for the Family
The baby – Weaning

There are many situations in which it is not possible to breast feed (for example, the baby so premature that is cannot yet suckle, or the mother suffering from infection that would be a danger to her child). Today, artificial substitutes for breast milk are vastly improved when compared with earlier versions but, from what I have said, you can understand that it is extremely difficult to create a product that matches the excellence of the human in all respects.

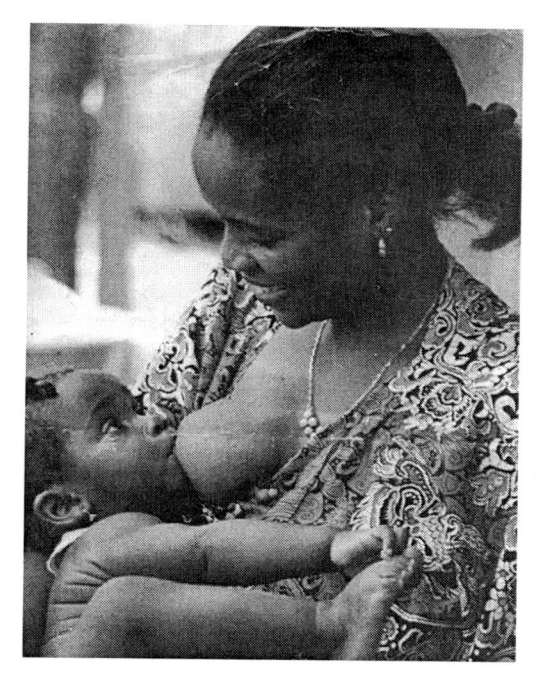

Unless there is no alternative, Breast is Best.

There is much argument regarding for how long breast feeding should be maintained. In some poorer societies, breast feeding may be continued for two or three years. This may be the consequence of foods' not being widely available. The evidence is that the child may suffer from various deficiencies. Some authorities insist that the optimum time is 4½ - 5 months, while others argue for longer; 8 - 9 months. What we do know for certain is that 'Breast is Best'. The breast fed child is healthier, less prone to gastrointestinal infection, is leaner, more compact and less likely to suffer upper respiratory infections, colds, chest infections etc.

When I was working in post-natal clinics, I could, whilst surveying the room from the doorway, pick out unerringly and by appearance alone, those babies that were breast fed and those that were not.

In later life, provided correct nutrition is maintained, there is less tendency to heart disease and other degenerative disorders, arthritis, age-onset (type II) diabetes, high blood pressure and in particular, obesity.

Weaning

In some primitive societies breast feeding may be maintained for two or three years because of economic needs in times of general food shortage. It also allows for the infant's acquiring teeth to deal with solid foods, prior to which the mother would begin to offer food which she herself had chewed to pap. Perhaps this would be similar to what our early ancestors would have done.

Today, the fashion in the developed countries is to breast feed for a shorter time – 9 to 12 months at most – and so to introduce solid foods earlier. Done properly, this could make good sense.

Earlier, I mentioned that as lactation proceeds so the constituents of the breast milk alter, some falling while others increase. What remains very low throughout is iron[1], so that over-long breast feeding, in the absence of any other food, may be

Nutrition for the Family
The baby – Weaning, and the growing infant

detrimental to the child. Iron is the essential component of haemoglobin, the protein in red blood cells which carries oxygen to all parts of the body and so ensuring proper function. Iron is also protective, playing a part in defence against infection and preventing damage by oxygen to the delicate essential fatty acids used in construction of brain and nerve cells. The use of B vitamins, also involved in the development of brain and nerve tissue, is determined by the presence of iron. This is important when you remember that the human baby's brain continues to grow for several years after birth. Iron is widely available in meats as well as vegetables, egg yolks and grains. For further information see the section on minerals.

Introduction of solid food should be gradual. Remember that, to the infant, all food is alien. At first only tastes should be offered (and be prepared for frequent spittings out!). The best foods are those that the parents (on a healthy diet) are eating. Babies can digest proteins very well – lean meat, fish free of bone, liver – all passed through a sieve and offered on the tip of a spoon will soon be accepted and digested without trouble. Similarly, all fresh green leafy vegetables, cooked soft (not 'al dente' to avoid the small baby's choking on lumpy food) and sieved are well tolerated.

What the small baby cannot digest is starch. Yet most advice given is to provide cereals, mashed potato and starchy fruits such as bananas. Eggs should be introduced cautiously, but only the yolk portion for the first 18 months, by which time the child should be able to deal with the white part. Even so, eggs should come into the diet infrequently; perhaps 2-3 times in a week. The reason for this is not because of the cholesterol content, but because some individuals can develop an intolerance to eggs when taken daily. Which means that the individual, older child or adult, can develop an allergy to the protein contained in the white portion of the egg and so a complete intolerance of eggs and any foodstuffs containing egg: with the loss of what is, after all, a valuable food.

During all this time, the baby will continue to breast feed, but as it begins to take more of its nourishment from solid food, water boiled and cooled, can be introduced gradually; not cows' milk or formula feeds. Fruits, at first sieved and in moderate amounts, can also be offered but not fruit juice or artificially conceived fruit drinks or squashes. Commercially produced 'pure' i.e. undiluted fruit juices are advertised as containing the juice of $3^{1}/_{2}$ lbs (1.5kg) of apples, or 15 oranges or 10 grapefruit per litre. Who in his or her right mind would eat that amount of fruit (in addition to other foods) in a day? Yet people do quaff these juices in excessively large amounts, without realising that they contain only part of the whole. If such juices are given to children, they should be given only occasionally, in small amounts well diluted in water and varied.

---

[1] *Low iron levels in the breast fed infant seem to favour the establishment of the beneficial, protective bacterial populations in the digestive tract and to deter the growth of pathogenic (disease-producing) organisms. As weaning proceeds the bowel flora alter and the need in the growing child, for iron, is increased.*

Nutrition for the Family
The growing child

Sugar should never in any form (remember 'sugar' includes honey, glucose, syrups and treacles) be introduced into the child's diet.

By the time the child has reached his or her second birthday, the food should include almost everything that the healthy eating parents themselves eat; one exception being mushrooms[1]. It seems that the tolerance to fungi develops later on, from 5-7 years of age.

The growing infant

In the less sophisticated societies and after weaning, children would partake of what their parents ate. They would be acquiring the knowledge, often hard earned, of what was beneficial and what was harmful: even lethal.

> **Eating as a family is important not simply for the acquiring of good habits of eating. It is an essential for development and nurturing the personality of the individual and the cultural health of the community. In the UK, a frighteningly high proportion (60%!) of children never sit as a family at table with their parents at a meal.**[2]

Overeating would not necessarily be a danger, because natural instincts would operate more easily. Physical activity would take care of any likely excess.

Note how animals (not necessarily including household pets, fed unnaturally) tend to eat to satisfy, but not to overeat.

Today, at least in 'Western' societies, we have to put in more careful thought as to what to give the children to eat. If the parents are following the healthy eating pattern of our ancestors, then the children can share their food. The present-day hazard is a cultural one; the presence of sugar and sweet stuffs, often offered as a 'treat' or a reward and hidden in soft drinks, plus the abundance of snack foods that encourage 'grazing'. True, the child weight for weight, has a greater demand for food than the adult. In the first place, it has a higher metabolic rate, its cells are dividing more rapidly as part of the process of growth. In the second place, it has smaller fuel reserves and needs feeding more often. Whereas in the relatively sedentary adult, breakfast is not vital despite all advice to the contrary ("you must start the day with a good breakfast") in the child it is essential.

Think of breakfast as being an agricultural meal; the farmer who rises at 5 or 6 o'clock in the morning, does 3 hours of hard physical work on an empty stomach and then has his substantial Break Fast. Those of us who tumble out of bed, only half-wakened and who would ply the equally half awakened stomach with food, would be courting trouble.

A child brought up to healthy eating and to enjoy the accompanying physical benefits, still has

---

[1] Many children can't digest mushrooms, without suffering gastrointestinal upset or vomiting until they reach 5-7 years of age.

[2] BBC Reith Lectures 2001

Nutrition for the Family

Hazards associated with breast feeding

the difficulty of resisting peer pressure. His or her contemporaries who are eating differently are apt to sneer at someone who does not conform. Such a child although having acquired a preference for healthy foods would also need support from parents and other responsible adults.

We humans are also born with such instincts. Unfortunately, in many societies we have also been taught to suppress them.

For example: a child, having eaten, might say "I have had enough" or " I am full up, I don't want any more." The adult might reply "you haven't finished what is on your plate. Finish it! Think of all the starving children in the world." The child might obey. If this is repeated often, soon the child would not recognise the signal telling it that is has eaten sufficiently and so become a chronic over-eater.

Another child being offered milk might say "I don't want it, I don't like it." The adult might not recognise that the child is expressing an instinctive reaction and is not misbehaving. Conditioned to think that milk is a good food for everyone, the adult will attempt to disguise it by turning it into a chocolate drink or other flavoured concoction and so, overriding the child's instinctive dislike – often creating a craving – and, unwittingly, doing it a harm.

Yet, some of our instincts continue to function. Imagine that you have been engaged in some strenuous activity in hot weather. Thirsty, you take a glass of water which you drink rapidly; then another. You may even begin to drink a third and then, all of a sudden, stop. Someone nearby might ask "Why do you stop, don't you like it?" whereupon you reply "Of course I do, but I have had enough". How do you know? have you been counting how many ounces or centilitres and think "I must stop"? No. Some other part of you has signaled "enough".

So, listen to your body. Even more importantly, allow the child to preserve its natural instincts and avoid the development of distorted tastes, e.g. sugar or wheat cravings and abnormal appetites.

It has long been known that wrong feeding is responsible for many illnesses that manifest in later life. Alarmingly, evidence is that young children, as young as 3-4 years of age, have been discovered to be developing atherosclerosis – fatty deposits in the arteries – precursor to heart disease. In the United Kingdom, we seem to be following the USA with increasing incidence of diabetes and obesity.

Hazards associated with breast feeding

From time to time, a worrying situation arises when a baby feeding from the breast becomes distressed. It may suffer colic, foul-smelling diarrhoea, skin rashes of varying severity and is in obvious discomfort and failing to thrive.

Brilliant research by Dr W.G. Whittlestone, anthropologist working in New Zealand, showed that if the mother were atopic[1] and, therefore, allergic to some food in her diet, commonly proteins in milk and grains, she could pass on that sensitivity, through the milk to the child, with consequent problems to the child. If the situation is recognised quickly and the mother takes steps to

---

[1] *atopy: hypersensitivity with an inherited tendency to acute allergic reaction, but without predisposition to any particular form of allergic reaction.*

Nutrition for the Family
Hazards associated with breast feeding

remove the offending item(s) (for example; milk in all its forms and milk products including all cheeses, cream, ice cream, yoghurt and any foods into which these are added) a complete return to normality occurs. Breast feeding can then continue without problems.

Late recognition, when the baby has lost weight, perhaps severely dehydrated because of diarrhoea or loss of fluid from weeping eczema, requires emergency treatment under the care of a children's specialist (paediatrician) and a switch to an artificial feeding formula, usually based on soya and fortified with omega 3 and omega 6 essential fatty acids. Curiously, cows' milk formula in which the milk has been subjected to prolonged high temperature, so altering the protein structure, does not always seem to produce the same reactions. Nevertheless, the disadvantage of cows' milk compared to breast milk and the individual's future health remains.

Most prescribed drugs can pass through the mother into breast milk and so affect the baby. Further problems include thrush, allergy and antibiotic induced diarrhoea.

Other hazards, the majority of which are man-made, abound. One is overconsumption by the nursing (and also the expectant) mother, of oily fish from contaminated waters. Whereas Atlantic salmon, tuna, swordfish and shellfish such as oysters and mussels are safe to eat, similar fish from Eastern and Asian waters often contain high levels of mercury; the result of uncontrolled release of mercury waste from manufacturing and gold mining[1].

The developing brain and nervous system of the fetus and of the infant at the breast are very vulnerable to poisons such as mercury, which tends to lodge in muscle and nervous tissue; resulting in subsequent mental and physical impairment.

Other poisons include many used in homes; especially insecticides, some cleaning agents and fungicides. On farms and in horticulture, use is made of weed-killers, fungicides, insecticides and rat poisons; the majority of which can find their way into the food chain.

All of the above may, at first sight be frightening. If you think about it however, you will see that, in the majority of situations, **most of these hazards are avoidable.**

These observation are meant to remind you always take note of the quality of the foods you choose to eat and, where possible, avoid the unnecessary use of chemicals in the home. Most advertised *"germ killers"* are more dangerous and no more effective than soap and water!

Lest you think that I am advocating widespread use of super killer chemicals capable of eliminating "all known germs", (as one sometimes sees advertised), perhaps some clarification would be helpful.

Contrary to the popular notion, the majority of bacteria and viruses are not harmful. In fact we

---

[1] *Doubts have been raised in some quarters regarding mercury contamination of farmed salmon in the UK. There is no evidence to support the idea that the farmed fish are any different in this respect from the free-swimming fish in the waters surrounding these farms.*

Hygiene
A diversion

humans live in a mutually beneficial partnership, symbiosis, with many of them. Relatively few are pathogenic, (i.e. capable of causing illness or death).

On the skin: colonies of bacteria exist on our skins, nourished by the oily, sebaceous excretions and dead skin cells. They form part of our defence against any potentially harmful organisms; bacteria or fungi. Experiments in which harmful bacteria have been applied to intact skin, have shown that, within minutes, no trace is left; only the usual 'friendly' bacteria can be cultured. These latter cannot be removed by normal washing; only by strong antiseptics, which should be avoided.

In the nose: specialised bacteria which can tolerate a high-salt environment, flourish to protect us from potential invaders; bacteria, viruses, fungi.

In the mouth: we carry a veritable army of organisms which can tolerate the enzymes and other secretions in the saliva. As you can imagine, the mouth is open (literally) to many intruders, good and bad.

In the vagina: Döderlein's bacilli (lactobacilli) tolerate a relatively acid environment and suppress the growth of other bacteria and yeasts.

Most of the bacteria that we swallow are destroyed, either by the strong acid that is present in the stomach, or by the strongly anti-bacterial bile and pancreatic enzymes present in the duodenum and in the jejunum; the first parts of the upper intestine. Some, however, can survive these hazards. Mostly they are the beneficial types, various lactobacilli and bifido bacteria; but more of that later.

> ### Here, may I make a plea?
>
> In a book about food, you may think this out of place, but some of the worst cases of severe gastro-enteritis, of life-threatening proportions, that I have seen in small babies have not been due to faulty feeding but to lack of hygiene: a baby's being handled by an adult who has used the WC without afterwards washing the hands; a worker in a crèche, where there are many small babies, changing the nappy of one and going straight from one to another, again without washing the hands each time. Infection in these situations spreads like wild fire. Toys that are (inevitably) thrown on the floor should be washed before given back to the child.
>
> **So, please wash (not scrub) your hands, again and again.**

First, I would like to offer you, in very shortened form, the lives and experiences (and the inferences we can derive) of two great men of medicine from the nineteenth century; Dr Semmelweiss of Hungary and Dr Lister of England.

The Tale of two cities
Semmelweiss (1818-1865)

Dr Ignatz Philipp Semmelweiss was a Hungarian physician, born in the city of Buda at the time of the Austro-Hungarian Empire.

Following graduation at the University in Vienna, he was appointed assistant professor in the maternity department of the hospital, under Professor Johann Klein.

At the time, the death-rate among parturient women from what was termed "puerperal fever", was alarming; rarely less than 5 and often more than 7 in a hundred. Between the months of October 1841 and May 1843 there were 829 deaths among a total of 5,139 women: a frightening 16%! Higher death-rates prevailed in the students' clinic compared with that of the midwives.

The death of a colleague from a dissection wound provided Semmelweiss with a clue to the answer. Each new patient coming into the already overcrowded ward would often have to occupy a bed with previously soiled linen. Students would come directly from dissecting rooms wearing contaminated clothing, usually kept specially for the purpose – a practice similar to that prevailing at the time among surgeons in Victorian England.

In May 1847, Semmelweiss instituted a new regime of cleanliness; properly cleaned wards, fresh, clean linen to each new admission and *careful hand washing* using chlorinated lime-water. The mortality rate fell from just over 12% in May to just over 3% by the end of the year and to $1^{1}/4$% the following year. Although applauded by many eminent colleagues, his own boss, Professor Klein, whether through jealously or vanity, vilified him to the extent that Semmelweiss was forced to leave Vienna. Perhaps his own irascibility, impatience and tactlessness may have contributed to the conflict.

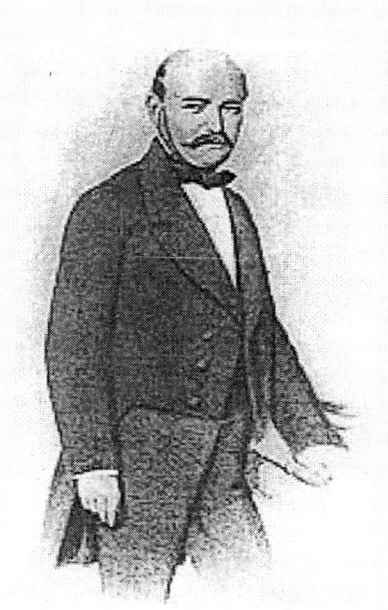

Fortunately, a year later he was appointed obstetric physician in the city of Pest where the same dreadful conditions prevailed. During his six years of office, by applying his methods, Semmelweiss succeeded in reducing mortality to less than 1%. The strain on him, however, led to his health's becoming so depleted as to compel him to rest and recuperate. On 20th July 1865, he was admitted to an infirmary for convalescence. It was a tragedy that prior to entry to this retreat, he had suffered a dissection wound in his right hand. On 17th August 1865, Dr Semmelweiss died of the very disease from which he had helped so many others to escape. Many of his detractors put about the story that his demise followed his being committed to an insane asylum. This was patently untrue.

The Tale of two cities
Lister (1827-1912)

Joseph Lister was an English surgeon, born in Essex in the east of England. He was educated and qualified in Medicine at University College, London and in October 1856, was appointed assistant surgeon at Edinburgh Royal Infirmary, Scotland. Five years later, he became surgeon at the Glasgow Royal Infirmary.

In spite of its being a new building, the deaths in the wards from what was called "hospital disease" (later, termed "operative sepsis") were appallingly high. Between 1861 and 1865 Lister recorded that 45-50 percent of his amputation cases died from septicaemia.

It was the work of the French researcher, Louis Pasteur, that alerted Lister. In 1865, Pasteur had suggested that microbes, living organisms in the air, could cause decay.

Lister already knew that "carbolic acid" (phenol) had been used previously in Carlisle, in the north of England, to treat sewage and that fields irrigated with the effluent had apparently become free of a disease-causing parasite affecting cattle. He immediately introduced a programme of anti-sepsis.

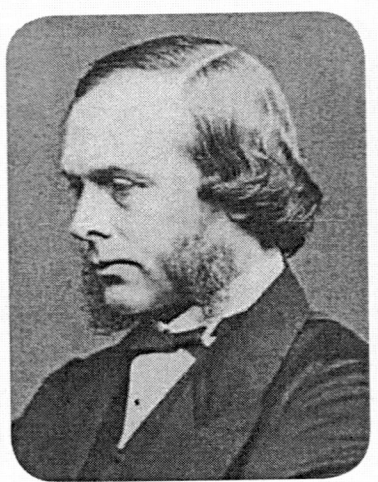

A dilute solution of carbolic acid was used to clean operating room floors, walls and tables; even spray the air. The patient was swabbed with the solution and surgeons had to wear a protective apron, similarly treated, over their (usually contaminated) clothing. Post-operatively, the wounds resulting from surgery were cleansed and dressed with solutions of carbolic acid. In 1867, Lister could declare that his wards had been free of sepsis for nine months.

In 1870, Lister's methods were used successfully by German surgeons during the Franco-Prussian war, thus saving many Prussian solders' lives.

A further advance in the prevention of spread of infection was made possible by the discovery in Germany, by Robert Koch in 1878, of steam sterilisation of instruments and dressings.

Lister gained much fame and honour, including a Barony and Order of Merit from Queen Victoria. His success stemmed primarily from his use of anti-sepsis – the killing of disease-causing organisms, but secondarily by use of asepsis – the removal of disease-causing organisms by simple cleaning methods; very similar to those initiated by Semmelweiss nearly two decades earlier.

These two men of genius, the one derided and denigrated, the other made famous and honoured, paved the way for the modern standards of cleanliness and the greater emphasis on asepsis rather than relying on anti-sepsis alone.

Hygiene
Public Health

It was at this time, in Victorian England, that a quiet revolution was occurring, which was to bring enormous benefit to the health of the nation; greater than anything so far achieved by the medical profession of the time.

In towns and cities, open sewers running in open gutters along the streets were being replaced by well-constructed underground tunnels, designed to take away the stinking and dangerous effluent of people and animals. Dry closets were being gradually replaced by water closets (WCs) also draining into the underground system.

Drinking water, hitherto drawn from rivers, ponds and wells and often contaminated, began to be distributed from water treatment plants. There it was filtered to remove solid contaminants and some micro-organisms, aerated to eliminate those microbes unable to survive when exposed to oxygen, and finally, treated with chlorine to ensure microbe-free transport of water through piping to the consumer.

At the time, cholera was endemic in the United Kingdom. As a result of the new measures, this life-threatening gastro-intestinal disease caused by faecal contamination, diminished and was, finally, vanquished. Britain became cholera-free. Similarly, a form of goitre associated with faecally contaminated water, not iodine deficiency, also disappeared.

It is unfortunate that despite all this evidence, education of the public did not and has not, even now, kept pace; is still sadly lacking. Facilities for hand-washing in public toilets in the UK only became universally available in the latter half of the 20th century. In contrast, in all the Middle Eastern countries that I have visited, washing facilities in toilets, both public and private, exist not only for washing one's hands but also the nether regions. The same cannot be said of most countries elsewhere.

There was an occasion whilst working in hospital in the 1950s when I was giving a lecture to a number of high-level business men, all highly intelligent and well-educated. The talk included the importance of washing the hands after using the WC because of the risk of infecting other people, especially babies in whom gastro-enteritic infection can be fatal. At the end of the lecture, I was approached by the Chairman of one of the companies who asked me in all seriousness, did I *really* mean what I said about the necessity of washing one's hands after using the WC?!

Today, we know that, worldwide, for people in the poorer, deprived communities, provision of clean drinking water and good sanitation is needed above all else. Given these, other problems such as inability to feed themselves become solvable.

Nevertheless, despite the privations they suffer, many impoverished people maintain good standards of personal hygiene. When I was in India towards the end of the Second World War, I was very impressed to note that most of the local inhabitants who were very poor and had very little water to use for all purposes, managed to attain a standard of personal cleanliness which was, in many cases, better than that of my own troops, who were more lavishly supplied.

Nutrition for the Family
– the growing child

Healthy children develop into healthy adults. They contribute to the well-being of their community, not so much in material prosperity as in mutual caring and contentment.

Sadly, the health of children in Britain has, during the past twenty five years, deteriorated. Chronic illness in children aged 5 - 15 years has more than doubled and in children under 5 years, more than trebled[1]. Sick children are likely to grow up into sick adults, with all the resultant misery - to say nothing of the resulting cost to the nation.

Most of this decline comes from poor nutrition. Surveys on children of school age 4 to 18 years show significant deficiencies in most of the essential vitamins and minerals[2]. School meals, once free for all (and which for most children would provide the main and often the only hot meal of the day) are now restricted to very few children from very poor homes. School meals have declined both in cost and nutritional content; in addition, most are so badly designed and, therefore, unattractive that almost half of those children entitled to free school meals reject them.

Conclusions [3]:

"School meals should be free like education."

1 The conclusion from the Survey of children aged 4 – 18 is that many more children need school meals than the children now eligible for free lunches.

2 It is cost effective to feed children in schools.

3 Free school meals would not only be a present benefit but would be an important investment for the future.

The present cost of providing all children with a free school lunch of increased quality would be between £2 and 3 thousand million sterling (House of Commons Committee Estimate) and compared to the £100 thousand million plus budget of the Department of Social Security, a small amount. So why not do it? The savings, not to say benefits, would be enormous.

The Solution

Recognition of what is natural and healthy eating is vital. Remember that you and I are the result of at least 4 million years of evolution. We are, therefore, adapted to eating a wide range of animal matter; meats, fish, eggs but also an even wider variety of green leafy vegetables, roots and fruits. We are not yet fully capable of handling sugar, starches and milk products.

Because children have a higher energy requirement, both for physical activity as well as for growth, they also have the need for more frequent and adequate meals both in the home and in school. Breakfast for the child is vital, whereas in the adult (unless physically active), it is not. Research among children in France indicates that meals eaten later in the day do not compensate for a missed or inadequate breakfast and proposes that

---

[1] *Living in Britain. Office for National Statistics.* London: Stationery Office

[2] *National Diet and Nutrition Survey; Young people aged 4 to 18 years* London: Stationery Office

[3] *Extracted from New Evidence on the Nutrition of British Schoolchildren and Conclusions for School Meals;* Margaret and the late Arthur Wynn: Journal of Nutrition and Health, 16, 2002

Nutrition for the Family
– the growing child

breakfast should constitute a quarter of the day's requirement. In these days of single parent families and working mothers, it would help if lunch at school were to be the main meal providing nearly half the total requirement.

For this to work, then you and I and my colleagues in the medical profession, the government, dieticians, must become aware of and to put into practice the principles that I have outlined. Financial cost is no excuse. It is perfectly possible to feed ourselves well and economically, but it requires intelligent thought and the need to break old habits and prejudices. Grains and starches and dairy products are cheap to produce and have a long shelf life and so offer convenience, but, with sugar, are implicated in the rise of physical and mental disorders and the related suffering.

The reward for our making the change would be a real improvement in health, both physical and mental, for ourselves and for our children, their children and their children's children.

Nutrition for the Family
– the teenager

The time of transformation from child to adult is both bewildering and exciting.

Besides the continuing growth in stature, is the development of the secondary sexual characteristics; appearance of axillary and pubic hair, with, in the male, beard formation and deepening of the voice; in the female enlargements of the breasts and arrival of menstruation (menarche). At this time, the body is subjected to a battery of hormonal changes including the rises in the sex hormones. Emotionally the individual is often hypersensitive and liable to severe mood swings.

It is at this time that we are most vulnerable to wrong feeding. If with our peers we are making a fashion of eating "junk foods" inadequate in vitamins, minerals and essential fatty acids and loaded with sugars, starches and the wrong kinds of fat, we are heading for trouble:

- Acne, especially, but not exclusively, in boys, together with appearance of blackheads and greasy skin;
- Menstrual problems in girls, painful and/or irregular periods, weight fluctuation due to fluid retention, mood swings;
- Eating disorders leading to uncontrolled excess (bulimia) or inability to eat (anorexia);
- Depression, having a chemical origin, not related to circumstances.

All of these conditions usually considered to be "part of growing up" are avoidable in the first place. Where they have developed, they are reversible by reverting to our "ancestral diet". Eating disorders may need additional expert professional help.

Nutrition for the Family
– the young man and young woman (20-50)

Watching children grow, it soon becomes apparent that growth seems to take place in little bursts. First there is a noticeable increase in height, followed by a pause while the child, previously seeming to become slimmer, now broadens. This is followed by another phase of growing taller and so on. This continues until the early teens when, coincident with the onset of puberty, there is a remarkable growth spurt during which the young person becomes rapidly taller. This continues until maximum height is attained – usually between the ages of 18-22 years. This is when the growing ends of the bones fuse, so that no further lengthening occurs.

What is not generally realised, is that growth is continuing and will do so until age 35-40. During this time, there is continuing increase in bone density and muscular development (a man of 40 years of age may not always be as supple but has much greater muscular power than he had at 20). Maturation, continuing development of other tissues and functions, takes place during this time.

A clue to this is in sleep requirement. Growth – and for that matter, repair – takes place best when one is asleep or resting.

The new-born baby sleeps almost through the twenty four hours, waking frequently for only short intervals. You see, the new-born baby is growing fast; the cells are dividing very rapidly. This growth rate, however, is slowing down and so a one year old child sleeps less than at birth because the body cells are dividing less rapidly. This continues through the years with the sleep requirements becoming less until levelling at around the age of 35-40. The only time sleep requirement will go up is during illness, after strenuous exercise and recovery from accident. If we were to plot the rates of cellular division over the years and the number of hours slept at each stage, we would get two identical curves.

It is at this crucial time, late teens and early twenties, that the young man and, nowadays, young woman embarks on a career, usually requiring long hours of work and study. Meals tend to become snacks, with consequent loss of essential nutrients, during a period when their importance is no less than at any time before. It is at this period that physical activity has also been allowed to slide. Remember that at this time you are still growing[1] and maturing and that many of you will be marrying and considering to become parents. Maintaining the ancestral diet and moderate regular exercise will assure your continuing good physical and mental health; virtually guaranteeing fit, lively, healthy, active old age. Besides which, establishing the habit of eating correctly as a family enables your children to grow up accepting this as normal and totally natural and so ensuring their future well-being.

---

[1] *This is why one's weight continues slowly to increase from the early 20s and levels off at the age 35-40, from when it should remain steady. The fact that in many cases it does not but continues to increase is a matter of life-style; lack of exercise, over-indulgence and/or incorrect diet.*

Nutrition for the Family
– the older man and older woman (50 plus until who knows . . . ?)

Requirements for older people are mostly similar to those of us all, but there are some differences.

Generally, there is a tendency to be less physically active[1] so that appetite is reduced with a consequent lessening of food intake. Added to this, in many older people enzyme activity and hormone production are lower, resulting in less efficient absorption of essentials in the food and consequent nutritional deficiencies. The resulting reduced energy levels lead to even less urge to be physically active, or even to trouble to prepare adequate meals – especially if one is living alone; a "Catch 22" situation.

People born in the United Kingdom prior to 1945-50 suffer a further disadvantage not shared by those born afterwards; tooth and gum diseases – products of poor diet and ignorance of correct dental care. The result: avoidance of foods that require chewing. For these people proper, modern professional dental care is essential.

All is not lost. Gloomy as the picture seems, it applies mostly to those whose diet has not matched up to the ideal. Nowadays we have the means to measure deficiencies, not only of vitamins and minerals, but also of hormone levels and digestive enzymes. Adoption of the ancestral diet with appropriate supplementation can produce surprising improvements and a restoration of well-being. On such a regime, the body's capability of normalising its own production of hormones and enzymes is restored. The restitution of vitality and therefore, physical activity is its own reward with a return of physical and mental well-being.

Growing older is a dream come true.

Illustration courtesy Bev Williams

You can't hear what annoyed you

You can't see what irritated you

And doing what you like takes much longer

---

[1] *In some countries there is a distinct difference in the amount of exercise undertaken by men and women. Some cultures seem to discourage, if not actively forbid for whatever reason, women to be physically active (at least in public). This inactivity can lead to osteoporosis, obesity and diabetes. In other cultures, the women do physical hard work while the men remain idle by comparison. The result is a shortened life span consequent on excessive wear and tear in a constitution functioning on an inadequate diet.*

Nutrition for the Family
– the vegetarian

The true vegetarian, or vegan, eats only food derived from plants; avoiding any of animal origin, whether meat, fish, egs or milk products. To me, this poses a problem. While recognising that for many, vegetarianism is a matter of culture, religious observance or philosophy, I can see no scientific evidence, neither anatomically nor physiologically, to justify it.

To be a truly healthy, active vegetarian can be difficult – especially in Britain.

Despite what I have just said, I have, for many years, had the good fortune to enjoy many different entirely vegetarian meals in different countries; creations of peasant people with little or no access to animal products. I can only admire the inventiveness and skills with which these people produce such delicious food and in such variety.

Why, in Britain, do we murder perfectly good vegetables and make them so unattractive and unpalatable (sometimes, in my experience, utterly revolting), is quite beyond my comprehension. Restaurants – even the most highly acclaimed – do no better. Any vegetables tend to be minimal in quantity, serving mainly as a decoration on the plate; not truly part of a meal. As a result, one is forced to *demand* adequate quantity and variety and a higher standard of preparation.

Vegetarian or not, you, Good Reader, should do more to discover what other people around the world do, with what is available, to make good food attactive as well as delicious.

While there is no doubt that the pre-human hominids were plant eaters, it is equally certain that, at least four million years ago, Man had evolved into a species deriving a high proportion of food from animal sources, but with a continuing dependence on a wide variety of foods of vegetable origin. This more concentrated diet, not only in energy content, supplied much "ready-made" material necessary for brain growth and development while lessening the time necessary for feeding. Herbivorous animals spend the greter part of their time seeking food: a horse, for instance, will spend sixteen to eighteen hours out of twenty four, eating.

You, the true vegetarian, must apply great thought in order to approximate to the "ancestral diet". Leafy green vegetables and roots pose no problem, but are low in energy and protein. Plants also vary in mineral numbers, needing fewer than we do. Similarly, plants vary in numbers of amino acids (the "building blocks" of protein), hence classed as supplying "Second-class" protein. Not true when you take care to maintain a wide variety of vegetables. Don't neglect the fungi which can supply an amino acid, lysine, commonly lacking. Any deficit in protein can be met with pulses – dried peas, beans, lentils – but beware! 100 grams (about four ounces) of dried product will provide 20 grams of protein; similar to that from the same amount of fish or meat. Cooked pulses will have absorbed water to four times their weight so that 100 grams now provide only 5 grams of protein. Ignorance of this fact can lead to serious protein deficiency.

Nutrition for the Family
– the vegetarian

Because of their carbohydrate content, pulses are also valuable to raise the energy density, which in the purely vegetable diet can be low.

Don't make the common mistake of many vegetarians who put too much emphasis on grains; it would put you at a serious nutritional risk.

As serious for the vegan is the difficulty in obtaining sufficient omega 3 fatty acids. We have already seen that, whereas the omega 6 essential fatty acids are present almost to excess, the omega 3 group, because of the lack of sea foods, is seriously low. With present knowledge, you can obtain the omega 3 EFAs from linseed (flax seed) and hempseed oils as well as from seaweeds, maritime plants (e.g. samphire) and nuts, including brazils, hazels and walnuts. Vitamin B_{12} is seriously lacking the the purely vetarian diet. to avoid the dangerous consequences of such a lack, I suggest you take a small supplement, preferably as part of a vitamin B complex formula.

It *is* possible to be a truly healthy, active vegetarian – with application of intelligence and knowledge.

Chapter 12

Functional Food

Functional Food
A new phenomenon

It would be appropriate, I think, for us to consider a relatively new phenomenon: functional food.

The term was first introduced in Japan during the mid-1980s and referred to processed foods which, besides being considered nutritious, also contained naturally occurring, not added, substances that assisted particular bodily functions.

These foods have since been renamed Foods for Specified Health Use (FOSHU). Originally, run under strict Government Control and testing, direction appears now to be entirely in the hands of the food producers. What seemed, in the beginning, to be a promising move towards improving the safety and quality of prepared foods, has degenerated into a free-for-all that certainly doesn't help the consumer.

In other countries, most notably the USA, interest has focussed more particularly on those naturally occurring foods which contain substances of known beneficial and/or protective influence.

Some examples:

Oysters and other molluscs are known to contain high levels of zinc. Zinc is particularly concentrated in the seminal fluid and zinc deficiency in men is linked (amongst other reasons) to diminished sex drive and to infertility.

Tomatoes, especially cooked tomatoes, are rich in lycopene, one of the family of carotenoids, which research has shown to be protective against cancer of the prostate; a gland in which, normally, lycopene is abundant. Lycopene alone, however, is not as effective in reducing the incidence of carcinogenesis as is whole tomato; implying that there are other substances present that work together. This protective effect is further enhanced when other vegetables are included in the diet: a tacit reminder that we are designed to eat *foods* and, unlike the Panda, not one but many different kinds – not nutrients alone.

Cruciferous vegetables, brassicas, include cabbage, kale, brussels sprouts, broccoli, cauliflower and contain a variety of enzymes and other chemicals. Consumption of brassicas has been shown to be related to reduced incidence of cancer; particularly of breast and colon. But beware: frequent, regular consumption of *raw* brassicas; notably cabbage (e.g. as coleslaw), is associated with interference with thyroid function, leading to a condition of hypothyroidism. The chemical responsible is destroyed in cooking, so removing the danger.

Garlic has been shown to reduce the incidence of stomach and colon cancers, has cholesterol lowering properties and is thought, therefore, to be cardio (heart) protective.

Citrus fruits are rich in a class of phytochemicals called limonoids. Limonene seems to be non-toxic and has been shown to be protective against a variety of human cancers.

Cranberry has been shown to have antibacterial properties and has been used effectively against urinary tract infections.

Functional Food

A new phenomenon

Linseed (flax seed) and Hempseed of all the vegetable oils, are particularly rich sources of alpha-linolenic (omega 3) essential fatty acid. It helps to reduce platelet aggregation (stickiness) and, therefore, spontaneous blood-clotting. Additionally, they contain phyto sterols[1] which may reduce risk of breast cancer

Tea, especially green tea, contains flavonoids which may protect against cardiovascular disease. Tea also contains polyphenols which, in high-risk populations, may protect against cancer.

Red grapes, red berries, red wine contain high levels of flavonoids, all of which have been shown to be strongly protective against heart disease. Another substance, resveratrol, has been shown to have cancer protective qualities.

All of foregoing are of plant origin, but there are also derivatives from animal sources.

Beef has already been mentioned as a source of conjugated linoleic acid CLA - in fact a group of isomers – found in the fat of ruminant animals, beef, lamb, venison etc. CLA has been found to be effective in preventing tumour formation in the stomach, colon and breast. Game meats are richer in CLA than farmed meats.

Fish, especially the oily fish and shellfish, are good sources of the polyunsaturated essential fatty acids of the omega 3 (n-3) group. These are known to be cardio protective, but as has already been mentioned, are also involved in the repair and maintenance of the brain and nervous system. Hormone production, mineral transport, birth of new cells to replace the old are all dependent on the omega 3 essential fatty acids.

These are examples of which there are, of course, very many more. While such knowledge can be useful, we must remember not to become obsessive about the components of any individual foodstuff. To think of mushrooms as only a possible good source of selenium leads to a restriction instead of expansion of variety of foods eaten. Besides which, eating would become a tedious, even boring mental exercise. True balance of nutrition can only be brought about, as said earlier, by *increasing* the varieties of *all* the different items in the diet; meats, fish, especially vegetables and fruits.

Remember that food should be source of pleasure and interest as well as providing the means for good health.

Why?

Do you remember my telling you about our sheep? How unhappy they were when on leys of one kind of grass only and how contented when in a field of old permanent pastures with a large variety of grasses and herbs?

When a patient tells me that he, or she, is "not interested in food . . . it is boring . . . I would rather take a pill than to be bothered to cook, or to eat a meal" (all of these things have been said to me; thankfully, not too often): Why should I worry? Because it is totally unnatural and indicative of a serious fault.

---

[1] *phyto sterols: biologically-active chemicals in plants.*

Functional Food
A new phenomenon

Think of it: if you go anywhere in the world, in any society – even the poorest – you will be offered hospitality in the form of food and drink and, where the need arises; rest. It is offered as a gesture of friendliness a source of pleasure – even survival.

If you invite people to your home, do you not do something similar with the intention of giving pleasure (and, in so doing derive pleasure yourself)?

Recently, I was standing at the edge of a small lake stocked with carp. In places, the water was violently agitated – even frothing – by the frenzied activity of dozens of fish. They were not fighting, mating or attempting to eat each other (the carp is, after all, a vegetarian), but feeding voraciously; fulfilling a biological need. *Without this inbuilt need and, therefore, the satisfaction derived from fulfilling it, no species could survive.*

Chapter 13

Obesity and Overweight & Relationship to ill-health

Obesity and overweight

If when I weigh myself the machine tells me that I am heavier than the books tell me that I should be, what do I tell myself?

That I am large boned?

Well built?

It is in my genes?

My height is far too short for my weight?

Or just plain fat?

Truly overweight (and this can lead to obesity) is multifactorial; many factors playing a part. Only one, however, is unarguably associated; wrong eating.

Our ancestral diet although containing energy-dense foods such as meat or fish, consisted largely of low-energy leafy vegetables, roots, fungi and berries. The diet in modern, developed societies is high-calorie, high-sugar, high-starch and relatively deficient in protein, correct fats – more so in green vegetables. Remember that, today, we are all far less physically active than were our ancestors.

The incidence of obesity is rising all over the world, in developing as well as developed countries. In the United Kingdom, it is estimated that 20%, in other words, one in five of the population is obese and, if that were not enough, 40% of the remainder are overweight. In the USA, over 60% of adults are overweight and in some states 50% are obese.

Obesity means an excessive amount of fat in the body. Most people who are overweight have become so because they have gained fat. Exceptions are to be found among those athletes who have increased

The weighing machine on its own is not a reliable guide to the fat content of the body.

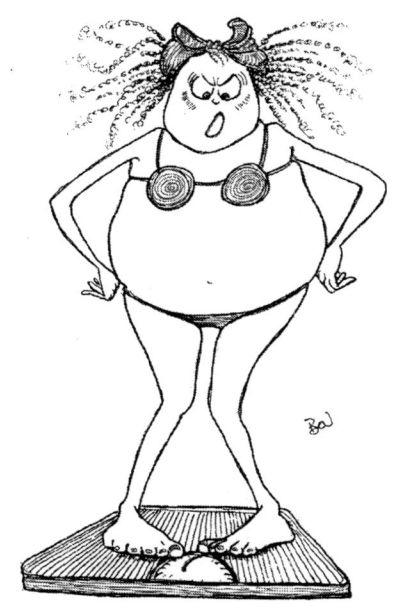

Don't be ridiculous

Illustration courtesy of Bev Williams © 2000

Obesity and overweight

muscular development. I know two brothers, professional strongmen, each 6 feet (about 1.8m) in height and each weighing 15 stone (about 95 kg). Each is 3 stones (19 kg) over the book weight, but without any excess fat. Such weight in this case should not be considered abnormal. Water retention with consequent increase in weight occurs in some women at a particular time of the menstrual cycle. It can also accompany some diseases involving heart or kidneys and is not an uncommon adverse result from some forms of medication.

abdominal fat, which is not revealed by the BMI. Waist measurements of more than 94 cm (37 inches) in men and 80 cm (31 1/2 inches) in women are associated with increased risk; over 102 cm (40 inches) in men and 88 cm (34 1/2 inches) in women, with greatly increased risk to health. Indeed the increased waist/hip ratio is a very strong indicator of risk for type II diabetes. It is a frightening fact that more children in the UK are ever younger becoming obese and destined to become obese adults. Children may not die from diseases associated with obesity, but adults most certainly do.

A more reliable, reasonably accurate, measure of fat content is the body mass index (BMI). This is calculated by dividing the weight in kilograms by the height in metres squared.

e.g. Weight 70 kg (11 stone) ÷ 1.752^2 (5 ft 9 in) = 23

According to World Health Organisation classification of overweight and obesity in adults

Classification	BMI (Kg/m2)	Risk of accompanying illness
Underweight	less than 18.5	Low, but risk of other clinical problems increases
Normal range	18.5 - 24.9	Average
Overweight	24.9 - 29.9	Mildly increased
Obese	30 and over	
	Class 1 - 30 - 34.9	Moderate
	Class 2 - 35 - 39.9	Severe
	Class 3 - 40 and over	Very severe

Although not 100% accurate, measurement of the BMI is a simple, easily done measurement of body fat if taken together with waist measurement. The latter gives some idea of the amount of intra-

As as been hinted earlier, a common consequence of obesity is development of type II diabetes. I also referred to 'age related' or 'age-onset' diabetes, meaning that it used to be seen to

Obesity and overweight
Liposuction – a warning

occur in overweight adults in their forties and fifties. Unfortunately, the term nowadays would be a complete misuse and type II diabetes is now occurring in children in their early teens.

That was the bad news. The good news is that obesity-associated risk of diabetes is essentially reversible. A combination of weight reduction by adoption of a healthy style of nutrition and appropriate physical exercise has proved to be very successful.

If you are overweight, adopting these simple measures brings additional benefits. The risks from type II diabetes are lessened, insulin sensitivity in the cells is restored and raised levels of blood pressure and cholesterol are normalised. Inflammatory markers (e.g. Homocysteine) and, therefore the risk of coronary heart disease are also reduced. All this adds up to increased mobility and a sustained general improvement in health and well-being.

A word of warning – Liposuction

This is a method of removing subcutaneous fat by mechanical suction through incisions made in the skin; commonly of the abdomen, buttocks and thighs, but also elsewhere and mainly for cosmetic reasons.

It is not a pleasant experience for the patient and, despite what some people will tell you, not without risk. It is a procedure, that in my opinion, should be adopted as an emergency where obesity is excessive and immediately life-threatening.

Certainly it is possible to remove considerable quantities of subcutaneous fat very quickly this way. Remarkably, none of the benefit of weight loss derived from correcting the nutrition together with appropriate physical exercise accompanies weight loss from liposuction. The body chemistry and, therefore, the attendant risks remain unaltered.

The only considerable reduction you could predict with certainty from treatment by liposuction would be in your bank account.

Obesity is rising alarmingly not only among adults but increasingly so in young children. In the United Kingdom, of 1.4 million people who have diabetes, around 90% have type II – so-called adult-onset diabetes, which is directly related to diet. It is thought that there are a further million undiagnosed cases. The numbers are predicted to double in the next 25 years. Already, type II diabetes has been recognised in British teenagers.

Food: the relationship to ill-health

Most illnesses in the civilised world – so called diseases of civilisation – are not the result of infection or accident. These metabolic or degenerative disorders stem from the body's inability to function properly; either from lack of essentials in the diet, or sometimes from excess causing imbalance, or from toxic (poisonous) substances present.

With correct management all of these conditions, even when well established, can be relieved; often completely cured.

Cardiovascular diseases

To name but a few, these include defects of the heart itself, leading to coronary disease and heart attack; hypertension (raised blood pressure) leading to heart failure and stroke; circulatory disorders, involving arteries and veins; atherosclerosis and narrowing of the former and weakening, varicosities and incompetence in the latter and ulcerations of the lower limbs; thrombosis (clotting) of the blood, involving heart, veins and brain.

The culprits most commonly associated are sugar (and thereby the starches which are rapidly turned into sugar during digestion) and excess salt which in some people is associated with raised blood pressure.

Gastrointestinal disorders

These include gastric and duodenal ulcerations (commonly associated with a bacterial infection – Helicobacter pylori); colitis (inflamed intestine) and irritable bowel syndrome (IBS) – this is not a diagnosis so much as a description – a blanket term for a variety of gastro-intestinal upsets where no specific disease has been identified. *It is estimated that one third of the British population is so afflicted.* Symptoms include anything from mild abdominal discomfort to severe, painful colic, erratic bowel functions and alternating constipation and diarrhoea. **Intestinal permeability** or "leaky gut" is the result of damage to the lining of the intestine allowing partially digested material to pass through. This damage is caused sometimes by infection, bacterial or yeast (e.g. Candida albicans) or parasites (e.g. amoeba), but commonly by inappropriate foods – mostly grains. **Constipation** is typically a disorder of civilisation and is a result of inadequate fibre in the diet i.e. a shortage of quantity and variety of leafy green vegetable matter. **Diverticular disease** is associated with constipation and is the result of inco-ordinate contractions in the bowel and excessive pressures generated when the colon contracts on an inadequate mass of bowel content causing small "blow outs" of lining through the muscular wall (diverticulosis). These blisters can at times fill with faecal matter and become inflamed and lead to the painful, sometimes dangerous condition of diverticulitis. Haemorrhoids in the veins of the terminal part of the colon, the rectum, result from the pressure developed in the effort to expel the motion.

Although irritable bowel syndrome is generally not considered to be *immediately* life-threatening, it

Food: the relationship to ill-health

should not be laughed off as being of no consequence. Effects can vary from moderately lowered vitality (and increased bad temper) to being severely crippling. The long-term effects are likely to be more serious and dangerous: increased risk of stomach or bowel perforation, haemorrhaging, stomach or colo rectal cancers.

The main culprits in gastro-intestinal disease are lack of sufficient quantity and variety of green leafy vegetables and fruits in the diet and the presence of 'alien' substances notably the grains; typically wheat in the UK, but other members of the grass family are often involved. Evidence exists that, in vulnerable people, milk and milk products cause similar damage.

Inflammatory bowel disease (IBD), which includes Crohn's Disease and Ulcerative Colitis, must not be confused with irritable bowel syndrome. The effects are more immediately severe and debilitating. They include severe abdominal pains, loose stools or diarrhoea with blood loss, raised temperature, tachycardia (fast heart rate) and anaemia. All need urgent professional attention, accurate diagnosis and treatment. Initially, severe cases require immediate medical support but, correct nutrition, often together with stress management can subsequently produce marked improvement and, if maintained, even complete remission.

The allergies and auto-immune disorders

These include asthma, hay fever (rhinitis) rheumatoid arthritis, multiple sclerosis, various forms of eczema, lupus, migraine and myalgias (muscle pains).

There is no one single cause for any of these conditions, but all are related to the failure of one or more of the immune systems. Stress is often an aggravating factor on an already weakened immunity and although diet has not been shown to be causative, an improvement in the diet will often produce amelioration.

Interestingly, in this age of super-cleanliness (some people appear to spend more on cleaning materials and germ killing substances than they do on food), it has been shown that children who are allowed from an early age to play out of doors in a garden or on soil and those who have grown up with animals, e.g. household pets such as dogs and cats or farm animals such as cows, sheep, horses etc., are less likely to develop hay-fever or asthma than those kept in a more sterile environment and whose immune systems have not been stimulated. So, should we be surprised to learn that certain intestinal worms have been used successfully to treat inflammatory colitis? (Perhaps this just adds weight to the argument that we are mistakenly, being *too* clean! see page 157.)

Cancers, which in our society appear to be on the increase in young people as well as those of advancing age, also indicate failures of the immune systems.

Cancer is a product of our modern life-style. It is unknown in people living in their primitive manner; the Inuit, the Kalahari bushmen, the Australian aboriginals. It is certain that even in a healthy body some cells become aberrant, but are swiftly dealt with by a watchful defence system.

Food: the relationship to ill-health

Modern man is being exposed to toxic materials. We know that tobacco is linked to cancers of the lung, colon and bladder. The air, particularly in towns and cities, is heavily tainted with petro-chemical, especially diesel vehicle exhaust fumes. In most households, chemicals are used for cleaning, some of which are dangerous to health. Fly killing sprays are related to nerve gasses and can damage the nervous system. In the garden, fungicides, weed killers and pest killers are all potentially dangerous.

Obviously, these substances should, if possible be avoided altogether or, at least, used with extreme care.

Nevertheless, healthy nutrition, with adequate intake of leafy green vegetables, enables the body to optimise its defences. Plants contain carotenoids, antioxidants and other phytochemicals which are protective. Some, such as are found in members of the cabbage family, can inhibit cancer growth.

The essential fatty acids of the omega 3 group have also been shown to be important. They include alpha-linolenic acid found in leafy green vegetables, but more abundantly in marine foods in company with eicosapentaenoic (EPA) and docosahexaenoic (DHA) acids.

Sports nutrition

This is a specialised subject and is outside the scope of this book. As mentioned in the section on vitamins and minerals, people engaged in high levels of physical activity may require higher levels of some items in their diet. This can only be done by expert supervision, requiring regular blood and urine analysis by specialist laboratories.

Some athletes require to develop muscles for speed or for strength or for stamina. Because the structure of the muscle cells is quite different for each requirement, management and training is also different. Only if the athlete in question is given completely expert and individual tuition, can he or she attain full potential without developing subsequent disabilities such as arthritis, cardiac and circulatory disorders, or immune deficiency; in short, a crippled and shortened life span.[1]

---

[1] See Bibliography, Exercise page 233

Chapter 14

Other illnessess associated with wrong feeding

Other illnesses associated with wrong feeding
Obesity

Obesity

Although the numbers of hungry people in the world have been lessening (6 million per annum since 1966), 14 million people in Africa are still starving, while in the USA 61 percent of the population are overweight. In the UK and developed countries 17-25% are obese and 40% of the rest are overweight.

The penalties of overweight are:
Diabetes Type II.

More than 90% of type II Diabetes is associated with overweight and obesity. It is associated with loss of sugar control and a lack of response to insulin. Constant high levels of glucose, with consequent imbalances of lipoproteins lead to deposits within the arteries (atherosclerosis) and high risk of myocardial infarction (heart failure).

Thickening of the lining of the blood vessels, particularly the carotid arteries supplying the brain, reduces the blood supply to vital organs. At the same time, the smaller arteries constrict causing a rise in blood pressure. Constriction of the smaller arteries (arterioles), seriously lessens the blood supply to the hands and feet, often to such a severe extent as to cause gangrene and to necessitate amputation.

Similarly, diminution of the blood supply to the retina of the eye – diabetic retinopathy, can cause blindness.

Raised blood pressure, as well as heart attacks, is linked to cerebro-vascular accidents; strokes.

Osteoarthritis, resulting from wear and increased joint pressure and diminished ability to repair is much more common when one is overweight.

Injuries from falls or accident are always more severe, and therefore, more dangerous.

Incontinence of urine in older people due to excess urine output associated with hyperglycaemia, is in fact reversible by correct eating.

Diabetic neuropathy is the involvement of the nervous system, partly caused by the impaired blood supply and by chemical interference of brain function.

Obstructive sleep apnoea, infertility in the male and the female as well as polycystic ovarian syndrome, gall bladder disease, are some of the other risks.

Happily much of this sad state of affairs is reversible, especially if action is taken as soon as any fault is recognised. A recent study at Oxford in England on nearly 700 people showed that increasing the proportion of vegetables and fruit in the diet was accompanied by a rise of antioxidant substances in the blood and a significant lowering of blood pressure.

Other illnesses associated with wrong feeding
Cancer, depression and other mental disorders

Cancer

I have already mentioned that 30-40% of cancers are now considered to be avoidable by eating correctly[1]. It is further estimated that with correct nutrition and the total avoidance of tobacco, the incidence of cancer world wide could be reduced by over 70%.

Remember cancer, like overweight, obesity, or type II diabetes, does not occur suddenly overnight. It is the result of deterioration taking place over a span of 20-30 or more years.

Likewise, any remedial measures will take a little longer, not 20-30 years, but a matter of some weeks, or months before a turn around and real benefit are experienced; in fact, in the opinion and experience of many it can be expected, not just hoped for.

Depression and other mental disorders

Like obesity, depression is becoming epidemic in so-called developed countries and in other parts of the world, especially where there has been a move towards the eating patterns prevalent in the USA and the UK.

The cause is certainly due to the change of eating patterns particularly in the last century. Today people are relying for sustenance on manufactured foods, which apart from being deficient in many important trace elements and vitamins offer a completely unbalanced supply of the essential fatty acids.

The essential fatty acids are comprised of two main groups; Omega 6 and Omega 3.

Earlier, when discussing evolution, I said that the Omega 6 fatty acids are common on land and that the Omega 3 fatty acids are most abundant in the marine environment. Members of the latter group are most importantly involved in the construction and function of the brain and nerve tissue. The two most prominent are Docosahexaenoic acid (DHA) and Eicosapentaenoic acid (EPA).

When our ancestors were evolving, particularly in the last 2 million years, they ate whatever wild or game, meat they could catch, fish including shellfish, occasional eggs, a wide variety of green leafy vegetables and berries; all rich in Omega 3 fatty acids. Omega 6 fatty acids would be present, coming largely from vegetables, roots and nuts. The balance between the two would be fairly equal, 1 to 1, 2 to 1, omega 6 to omega 3.

Today because of the dramatic change in our food, manufactured and with a reduced fish intake, especially the oily fish, the ratio has been grossly altered. Present day diets contain 15-25 times as much of omega 6 compared to Omega 3. Taken together with mineral and vitamin deficiencies, such imbalance can have serious effects on the brain chemistry and, therefore, mood and mental function.

---

[1] *Sir Richard Doll of Oxford University, England, is famously renowned for his verification of the connection between smoking and lung cancer.*
He also investigated the occurrences of different cancers in various countries. In 1968 he published the results of his findings and his conclusions; that 30-70% of all cancers related to food.

Other illnesses associated with wrong feeding
Chronic sickness

Research around the world shows a strong correlation with a nation's incidence of depression and reduced consumption of sea foods. Evidence includes other mental disorders including homicide, suicide, bipolar disorders (manic depression) and post-natal depression.

Where Western diet, including manufactured food, invades a culture where depression was low, the rate of depression rises accordingly: together with an increase in criminal and antisocial behaviour.

Chronic sickness and proneness to infection

The answer once again would appear to be in your hands. Eat more fish, including the oily fish. Increase the variety of green vegetables and roots. Eat lean meat, including game meat[1], occasional eggs and fresh (not salted) nuts[2] in shell and, of course, fruits in variety. Avoid the starchy foods, sugars, and all dairy products. In the kitchen use only a neutral, stable oil such as virgin olive oil.

General unwellness, vulnerability to infections, colds, influenza, sinusitis, bronchitis, gastrointestinal upsets have increased over the past 25-30 years. Recently recognised disorders such as myalgic encephalopathy, chronic fatigue syndrome, irritable bowel syndrome, have mushroomed; particularly in late teenagers and young middle aged people. The decline continues. Yet every situation is correctable with the re-installment of the right nutritional programme. Even the more crippling forms of colitis including the ulcerative form respond, but require professional help and guidance.

---

[1] *Game meat includes venison, wild boar, rabbit, hare, partridge, pheasant, grouse, wild duck and many more.*

[2] *Nuts would include walnuts, filberts or hazel nuts, pecans, cashews, pine, pistachio and others.*

Chapter 15

Food Allergy

Food Allergy

Food allergy is a subject that commands increasing attention. It was first brought to the public eye in the 1940s by Dr Theron Randolph of Chicago University, USA[1].

Genuine food allergy certainly does exist and it is, perhaps, no surprise that the foods that have appeared since farming began (e.g. milk, milk products and grains) are the most commonly involved. Reactions occur, but less frequently to other groups such as the belladonna family (aubergine, capsicum, potato, tomato) and some of the pulses. There is a rarer response in some individuals to pre-agricultural-type foods: some meats e.g. pork, certain fish and even herbs, such as artimesias (tarragon) and mints.

In my opinion, many of the latter are acquired:
- in the womb – sensitivity conveyed from an affected mother;
- after birth, either as sensitivity from the mother through her milk, but frequently because of gastro-intestinal infection – the result of lack of basic hygiene by people handling the baby;
- from infected food material, meat, fish, vegetable – even water;
- from use of improperly reared/hybridised animals – notably, in the UK, chicken and pork;
- from too early introduction of certain foods, e.g. white of egg.

---

[1] An Alternative approach to Allergies
Theron G. Randolph, M.D. and Ralph W. Moss, PhD
ISBN 0-690-01998-x

Nevertheless, true food allergy is much less common than is generally supposed.

How can this be so? I and many of my colleagues frequently encounter patients who react badly to almost everything they eat. For many years, I was puzzled and at a loss to understand what was happening. The reality is that many of these people are not truly allergic, but have suffered damage to the intestinal tract, which is allowing partially digested material to pass through the intestinal wall and into the system.

Think of the intestine as being a tube perforated with tiny holes. Now, imagine that – equipped with super-microscopic vision – you can see a molecule of protein, about the size of football. During digestion, this is reduced to smaller units, polypeptides, in size resembling that of a grapefruit. Each polypeptide is, in turn, broken down to smaller units, peptides, the size of a golf ball. Finally, these are reduced to the even smaller amino acids – in imagination, the size of a pea – which can pass comfortably through the holes in the intestinal lining and so into the blood flowing to the liver. That is how it should be and all is well.

When the intestinal lining is damaged, either by infection or by inflammation evoked by unsuitable foods, the little holes become enlarged and allow the "golf ball" or even the "grapefruit" to pass through. The body reacts immediately to this foreign invasion and symptoms develop suggestive

Food Allergy

of allergy, ranging from acute abdominal distress, to breathing problems, rhinitis, skin eruptions and general malaise. The condition is described as intestinal permeability, or "leaky gut", for which, thankfully, there is a specific diagnostic test.

Fortunately, once the cause has been identified, such damage can be repaired with the elimination of all symptoms.

How?

- Establish *and maintain* correct nutrition for the individual. If a true allergy exists, exclude *completely and for all time*, the offending item. I do not think that masking reactions by attempts at vaccination or by use of suppressive medication is wise and may, in the long term, prove harmful.
- Eliminate any infection that may be present, e.g. Helicobacter pylori in the stomach; yeast overgrowth in the intestine.
- Restore the bowel flora by oral administration of human-compatible strains of lactobacillus acidophilus and Bifidobacterium bifidus in adequate amounts.

Not every instance of abdominal upset can be laid at the door of intestinal permeability. Nevertheless, there is a very useful test (PEG 400) that can help the investigator. It is devised and performed by the Biolab Medical Unit *(see bibliography)* and involves the use of a liquid whose many components, have different molecular sizes; polyethylene glycol, related to anti-freeze. A measured amount is given to the patient to drink and subsequently urine is collected for six hours, the volume measured accurately and a sample taken for analysis.
The charts below and opposite show how such identification can be made.

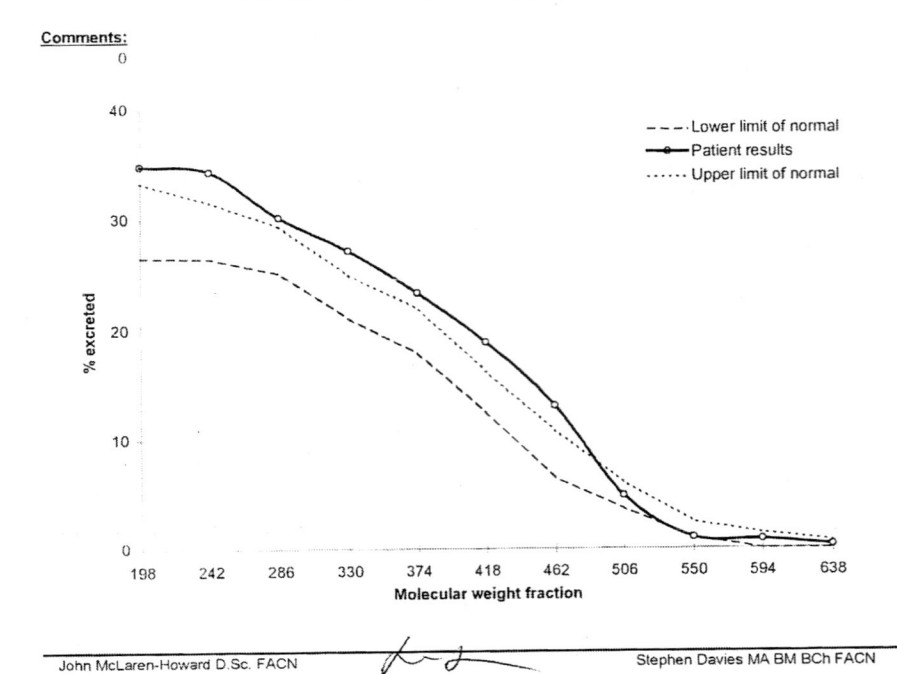

Comments:

Here is an abnormal result in a child age ten years.

There was a history of increasing abdominal pain and discomfort, but no obvious pathology was discovered, such as appendicitis, nor was there any evidence of infection or infestation such as worms. the damage had accrued from intolerance to milk and milk products such as cheese and yoghurt. Elimination of these allowed healing to occur and cessation of symptoms.

John McLaren-Howard D.Sc. FACN   Stephen Davies MA BM BCh FACN

Food Allergy
Intestinal permeability testing

Comments:

[Graph 1: Abnormal result — % excreted vs Molecular weight fraction (198–638), showing patient results above upper limit of normal across most of the range.]

John McLaren-Howard D.Sc. FACN   Stephen Davies MA BM BCh FACN

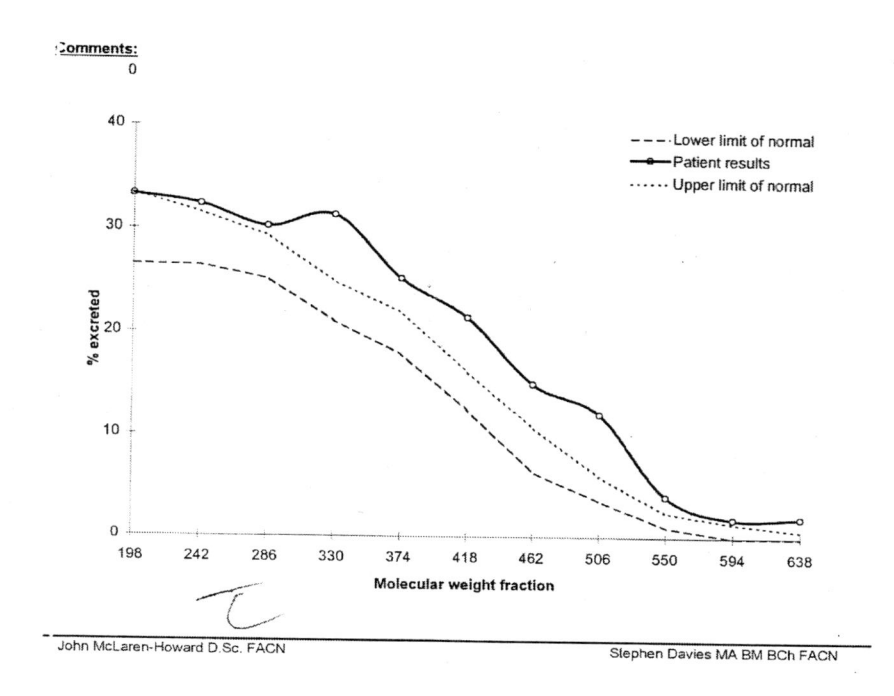

Here is a totally abnormal result in an adult, showing that over-large molecules were passing through the intestinal wall and into the system, finally being excreted into the urine.

The causes in this case were due firstly to intestinal yeast overgrowth following antibiotic treatment for a chest infection and secondly, to a marked intolerance to wheat.

Elimination of both causes produced clinical improvement.

Comments:
Normal gut permeability to PEG.

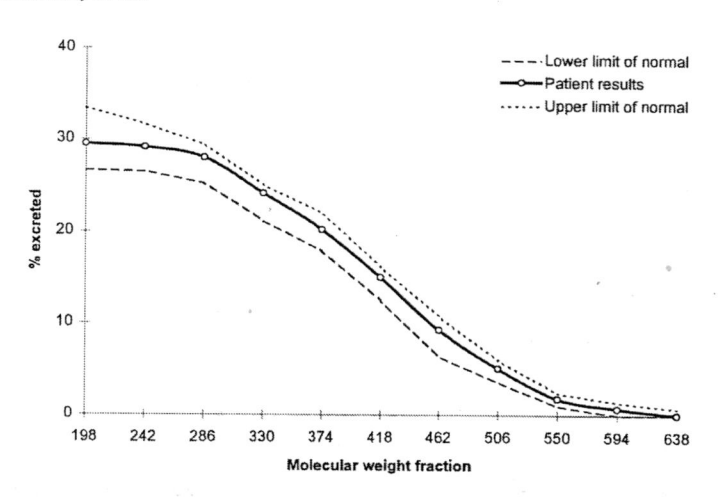

[Graph 2: Normal result — % excreted vs Molecular weight fraction (198–638), showing patient results within normal limits.]

McLaren-Howard D.Sc. FACN   Stephen Davies MA BM BCh FA

The normal result shown in a subsequent test made on the same adult above after the causes of intestinal permeability were removed.

Chapter 16

Cancer – some thoughts

Cancer – Some thoughts

At conception, the male sperm cell fuses with the female cell, the ovum. This impregnated cell – or stem cell – then divides to produce two identical daughter cells, which in turn produce four grand daughters. Further division produces eight, then sixteen, thirty two and so on ending up by producing a mulberry-like globular mass of apparently identical, undifferentiated cells – the morula. Suddenly, a change occurs when the cells of the morula form two quite different layers and mysteriously an order is imposed. In this new organisation, one cell will in the future become a skin cell, another a brain cell of a certain kind, yet another a muscle cell. Once this order is imposed, the course of each cell is fixed so that liver cells produce only liver cells, kidney cells produce only kidney cells and so on.

When you suffer an injury such as a cut of the skin, a series of local chemical reactions occurs to stimulate the adjacent tissues to heal the breach. New cells of necessary type, skin, blood vessel, nerve, muscle are rapidly produced. The edges of the cut are brought together and then everything stops, leaving the wound neatly healed. Have you ever considered how this happens? What monitors the repair activity and prevents its continuing unchecked? The body is equipped with hundreds of such necessary control mechanisms, which usually function extremely well. Even so, among the millions of actions within the body, there is always a situation where a cell or cells may go out of control. In fact, I am sure that while I am writing this a hundred such events are taking place in me and are being automatically corrected.

Cancers, of which there are as many kinds as there are different kinds of cell in the body, occur when such cells revert to the primitive state and begin to multiply without control. In the vast majority of cases, the causes are environmental. Work done by the World Health Organisation and the International Cancer Research Fund reveals that thirty percent of all cancers are due to faulty nutrition (other research suggests over forty five percent) and that a further thirty to thirty five percent are linked to tobacco smoking. **In other words between sixty and eighty percent of all cancers are potentially avoidable by paying attention to these two factors alone.**

Other environmental causes:

natural:

nuclear radiation from radon gas in some granitic soils; ultra-violet radiation from over exposure to sunlight; parasitic infections, including viral and fungal infections, amoebiasis, flukes and worm infestations.

Man-made causes:

radiation; nuclear radiation from x-rays (diagnostic and therapeutic), contamination from nuclear power plants, so-called "soft x-rays" emitted from television and some types of computer screens,

Cancer – Some thoughts

ultra-violet radiation from sun beds, electro magnetic radiation from high voltage power lines, excessive unscreened household electrical wiring, mobile telephones and microwave cookers.

chemicals; it is estimated that by the end of the twentieth century over one million chemical compounds have appeared that have never previously existed in nature. Some have been produced for military purposes, some for industrial use but include several thousands that are added to prepared foodstuffs in the form of artificial flavourings, colourants, texturisers, perfumes, taste-enhancers, preservatives, moisturisers, "brighteners" to produce a sparkle in beers. Most of these are of dubious merit other than to make inferior quality foods to be attractive, but some are frankly harmful (e.g. artificial colourants capable of producing allergic reactions including asthma and behaviour problems). Other chemicals include formaldehydes in toiletry and cosmetic preparations and glues used in chip board manufacture; solvents and driers in paints; oestrogens in pesticides and plastics; asbestos, previously used as an insulating material and in the manufacture of roofing material.

Genetic causes:

these form the smallest category. For instance, less than ten percent of all breast cancers can be attributed with certainty to inheritance.

Whether a person develops cancer – and for that matter, is able to overcome it – depends on the body's ability to defend itself. Do you remember that I said that food is not just a fuel, but a supplier of all the materials necessary for the body to repair and to maintain itself? Among these are nutrients that are essential for the proper functioning of the defence systems[1]. Here we have a possible reason why only some of the people living in particular circumstances develop some form of cancer while others do not. For instance, it has been shown that adequate supplies of vitamin D (in association with vitamin A)[2] can prevent the run-away division of cells typical of many cancers and can even cause them to destroy themselves (apoptosis) or revert to normal behaviour (redifferentiation). Other defence systems use selenium together with vitamin E, the carotenoids, vitamin C, all of which enable the body to manufacture specific materials with which it can protect itself even in hostile conditions.

What should you and I be doing to ensure that this is so?

Use as wide a range of (mainly) leafy green vegetables – raw and cooked – including where possible marine plants (seaweeds) and maritime plants e.g. samphire, asparagus. Where possible, use only organically grown vegetables. Similarly, fruits should be used in variety. In both cases consider *quality* and *variety*, not vast quantities.

[1] All of these materials – phytochemicals – *can only be derived originally from plants.*

[2] see section on vitamins : vitamin D *pages 109 & 110.*

Cancer – Some thoughts

Man has evolved to become dependent on animal sources as part of his food. Fish of all kinds, including the oily fish and shellfish are important as are good quality lean meats – especially wild or game meats of all kinds, including offals.

Listen to your body. It will tell you if a particular item – meat, fish egg or a particular vegetable – is causing discomfort or distress.

Where possible, avoid three items that have appeared in the diet since the advent of agriculture, viz. sugar (including honey, treacles, syrups) milk and milk products and grains.

Despite being on the increase, the majority of cancers are preventable. The answers are in your hands: correct your nutrition and improve your lifestyle as I have outlined in this book. Additionally, two specific items are known to be actively protective:

1. The Omega 3 long-chain essential fatty acids derived mainly from marine foods (not linseed). Unfortunately, there is such a gross imbalance in the modern diet between omega 6 and omega 3 essential fatty acids – upwards of 15 to 1 instead of 1 or 2 to 1 – that I have been reluctantly forced to admit the need for some form of supplementation of omega 3 essential fatty acids as well as dietary correction to redress the balance.
2. The Lactic acid bacteria (many different strains of Bifidobacteria and Lactobacilli) important species forming part of the bowel flora which populate the healthy digestive tract. They are damaged by faulty nutrition (see notes on prebiotics) and by antibiotics. In many people, bacterial dysbiosis (imbalance) has been present since birth; induced by malnutrition of the mother during pregnancy.

Recolonisation of the digestive tract is possible, but out of what has become an industry, only a very few laboratories[1] are producing strains of bacteria which are human compatible and sufficiently vigorous to survive in the human gut. Most so-called probiotics are of animal derivation and pass through without establishing themselves. Lactobacillus bulgaricus in yoghurt behaves similarly.

---

[1] Two reliable producers in the UK assessed by an independent body: Biocare Ltd, Kings Norton, BIRMINGHAM B30 3NU • UK
Blackmores UK Ltd, COLNBROOK, Buckinghamshire SL3 0PD • UK

Chapter 17

Examples of different foods

Some Examples of Different Foods

Vegetables

1 Vegetables

On our planet, Earth, *all* life that is based on the element carbon, is derived from plants.

Animals of all kinds depend on the vegetable world for materials that they cannot by themselves obtain: minerals; most vitamins; amino acids and simple proteins; the essential fatty acids (Linoleic and alpha-linolenic) as well as other vital chemicals. **Vegetables in our food include:**

Leafy green vegetables: some examples;

Artichoke (globe), asparagus, green beans in pod (young broad beans, dwarf French, pole and runner), leaf beet (chard), broccoli, burnet, brussels sprouts, cabbage, calaloo, cardoon, cauliflower, celery, chicories (endives), corn salad (mache, lambs' lettuce), claytonia (winter purslane, miner's lettuce), mustard, onion, parsley, green peas and peas in pod (mangetout, sugar snap), purslane, rocket (roquette, rucola), sea kale, shallot, sorrel, spinach, New Zealand spinach, watercress.

Fungi: Include a very wide range of wild and cultivated mushrooms, toadstools and truffles. Contrary to popular opinion, most fungi are nutritionally very superior. Many are rich in lysine, an amino acid which is lacking in many vegetables. They also contain significant amounts of protein and some valuable trace elements.

Roots and tubers: Artichokes (Jerusalem), beetroot, carrot, celeriac, ginger, mangel, parsnip, potato, radish, salsify, scorzonera, swede, sweet potato, turnip and yam.

Pulses (legumes): Dried broad (Fava) beans, other various dried beans, peas, lentils, "monkey nuts" (peanuts).

"Fruits" regarded as vegetables: Aubergine, avocado, capsicums (sweet peppers), courgette, cucumber, okra (bhindi, ladies' fingers), marrow (squash), peppers (chilli), pumpkin, tomatillo (physalis exocarpa), tomato.

Nuts and seeds: Almond, Brazil nut, cashew, chestnut, cob (hazel), macadamia, "monkey nut" (peanut – not a true nut, but a legume), pine, pistachio, walnut and coconut.

Seeds: include caraway, poppy, pumpkin, sesame and sunflower.

Many British readers will think **he's forgotten rhubarb**. I had indeed, until I was reminded. I choose, however, deliberately to **omit** it, with reasons:
- rhubarb is a plant with leaves rich in oxalic acid and which are very poisonous[1]. Although the stems which are eaten contain much less[2], some susceptible people can develop oxalate stones in the gallbladder and kidneys; both conditions can be dangerous and excruciatingly painful;
- of greater hazard generally, in Britain rhubarb is regarded more as a fruit than a vegetable; being used as a dessert. The highly acidic nature of the stalks demands cooking with large amounts of sugar or syrup and often finished with a "crumble" consisting of more sugar, breadcrumbs and fat – a lethal combination. Finally the accompaniment is a custard made from cornflour, artificial flavouring and colour, milk and more sugar!

[1] *During the First World War, 1914-1918, there developed in Britain an increasingly very severe food shortage, amounting almost to famine. Many people died as a result of eating rhubarb leaves as a substitute vegetable.*

[2] *Sorrel, used in salads and soups, also contains oxalic acid but is consumed less often and in smaller amounts; strawberries and spinach also.*

Some Examples of Different Foods
Vegetables and Animals

Fruits include: Apple*, apricot*, banana*, blackberry, black (and red and white) currant, blueberry, cape gooseberry (chinese lantern, physalis edulis), chinese gooseberry (Kiwi fruit, achtinidia chinensis), cranberry, cherry, date* elderberry, fig,* gooseberry, grapefruit, grape*, lemon, lime, mango, medlar, melon, mulberry, nectarine, orange, papaya, passion fruit, peach, pear, pineapple*, plum*, quince, raspberry, strawberry, tangerine, New Zealand tree tomato.

* often preserved by drying.

Grains include: Barley, buckwheat*, maize, millet, oats, quinoa*, rice, rye, wheat, wild rice.

* not members of the grass family; graminae.

Vegetable oils and fats: Almond, avocado, blackcurrant[1], borage[1], candlenut, castor, cocoa[3], coconut[3], corn (maize), cotton seed[4], evening primrose[1], grape seed, hempseed[2], linseed[2] (flax), mustard, olive, palm[3], peanut, rape[4], safflower, sesame, soybean, sunflower, walnut.

[1] used therapeutically as sources of omega 6 essential fatty acids.

[2] used therapeutically as vegetable sources of omega 3 essential fatty acids.

[3] saturated fats.

[4] preferably to be avoided; potentially toxic.

Most of these oils are unsaturated to a greater or lesser extent. They are highly unstable and easily degraded, primarily in the manufacturing process and, subsequently, on exposure to air (oxygen), heat and light. The result is a physical distortion and production of what is called a *trans* fatty acid, which can cause severe, even dangerous, interference with lipid metabolism; blocking important chemical processes and behaving in many ways worse than an excess of saturated fat. Such trans fatty acids also are to be found in margarines, other butter substitutes and manufactured foods; cakes, biscuits, crisps etc.

The safest oil for all culinary use is virgin (cold pressed) olive oil: other oils should, if possible, be avoided. Oils such as sesame and walnut, used for flavouring, should be kept cooled, sealed in dark glass or opaque containers and not heated.

2 Animals

All are good sources of "first-class" protein (containing all the amino acids needed to form any kind of new protein for the consumer); essential fatty acids (omega 3 in particular); vitamins A, D, E, K and all the B vitamins, including B_{12}; minerals, including iron, calcium, phosphorous, selenium and zinc.

Meats in our food include:
Mammalian
  Wild/game: deer, gazelle, hare, hedgehog, rabbit, badger, coypu, squirrel, wild boar.
  Marine: dolphin, whale.
  Domesticated: beef, camel, goat, lamb, pork.
Avian
  Wild: blackcock, capercailzie, duck, grouse, partridge, pigeon, pheasant, quail, snipe.
  Domesticated: chicken, duck, goose, guinea fowl, ostrich, quail, turkey.
Reptilian/amphibian
  Mostly wild: frog, crocodile, lizard, salamander, snake. (In many societies, grubs, insects and snails are equally important).

Some Examples of Different Foods
Fish and Eggs

Consumption should not be limited to muscle meat. Offals, often today sadly ignored, are valuable sources of important nutrients: liver; lights, or lites (lungs); heart; kidney; sweetbreads (pancreas and thyroid glands); tripes; intestines (chitterlings – English, andouillettes – French). Unfortunately, because of the present fear of spongiform encephalopathies, not brains!

Fish

All fish are as valuable as meat, being good providers of **proteins, vitamins minerals and essential fatty acids.**

The oily fish are especially rich in the omega 3 essential fatty acids and in the longer chain omega 3 fatty acids, eicosapentaenoic and docosahexaenoic, so important in the formation and functioning of the brain and nervous system.

Included among the oily fish are: albacore, eels, herring, mackerel, octopus, pilchard, salmon, sardine, shark, skate (ray), sprats, squid, sturgeon, swordfish, trout, tuna.

Shellfish are also valuable both in nutritional content and in supplying trace minerals, such as manganese, selenium and zinc.

Included among shellfish are:

Crustaceans: crabs, langoustines, lobsters, prawns, shrimps.

Molluscs: clams, mussels, oysters, scallops.

Gastropods: limpets, whelks, winkles.

Rich sources of protein and essential fatty acids are to be found in *fish roes* of such fish as cod, herring, salmon, sturgeon and many others.

Eggs

Eggs from all kinds of birds constitute a valuable food.

Apart from children under two years of age, (who tend to react against the white part) eggs are well tolerated by most people and are a valuable source of protein, the B vitamins including B_{12}, carotenes and minerals including calcium, iron, manganese and zinc. Cholesterol is present as is lecithin (an emulsifier which, among other things, helps to prevent the formation of obstructive plaques in the blood vessels).

It is wise not to take eggs too frequently (i.e. daily), not because of the cholesterol content, but because some people can acquire intolerance – even allergy; which would be a shame to lose such a valuable food. So, remember that is is not the *number* of eggs eaten but the *frequency*. In other words, you could have a four egg omelette twice a week, but not an egg every day.

> While on the subject of eggs: a further piece of nonsense, which appears to have originated in the USA, advises people to discard the yolk and use only the white part in an omelette or to eat with their grilled bacon. This ill-conceived advice seems to stem from a phobia for consuming fats and cholesterol containing foods; the same misconception that led the American Medical Association and Federal Food and Drugs Administration to advise their countrymen and women to adopt a low protein, low fat and high carbohydrate diet. The disastrous consequence has been that they are all fatter and are suffering an epidemic of obesity with all the attendant ills.

Chapter 18

The Blood type groups

The Blood type groups
Features in common.

Meat: only type A shows less tolerance to most meats. The others benefit but less than type O.

Fish: all types benefit, but only type O seems to be able to deal with all molluscs and crustaceans.

Eggs: all types tolerate and benefit (with individual exceptions within each blood group).

Grains: Wheat can upset all blood group types. Other grains vary greatly in acceptability. Blood group type O seems least able to manage any grains without eventual damage.

Leafy green vegetables: are of benefit to all blood groups. The exceptions are members of the belladonna family, which are not always well tolerated by blood group types O and A. There are always individual intolerances to a particular vegetable in any blood group.

Fruit and berries: benefit all blood group types.

Roots, tubers and fungi: are generally of benefit and well tolerated. The exception is the potato (a tuber) which, because of its starchy nature and high glycaemic index should, in a mixed diet, be avoided.

Legumes: are not well tolerated by blood group type O. Other groups can use them, but with individual variations.

Maritime plants, marine vegetables and seaweeds: all without exception are well tolerated and beneficial to all blood groups.

Nuts and seeds: most are well tolerated. Some such as walnuts and linseed can contribute valuable omega 3 essential fatty acids which are deficient in a vegetarian diet. There may be intolerance to sesame and sunflower seeds in blood group types B and AB.

Herbs: benefit all blood group types. There are always individuals in any blood group with antipathy to herbs of a particular family, e.g. mint.

Milk and milk products: Blood group type O is the least tolerant of milk and milk products. Remember that milk varies from species to species; is designed for the infant of that particular species and avoided subsequently. Some altered (fermented) milk products such as cheese or yoghurt can be used (with caution) by some individuals of blood group types A, B and AB.

Fats: those existing in lean meats, fish, shellfish and leafy vegetables are suitable and acceptable by all blood groups. For culinary purposes, the only truly safe one is cold-pressed (virgin) olive oil.

Sugar: added sugar is dangerous for all blood group types and, therefore, taboo.

Starch: human beings are not equipped to deal with raw starch such as that derived from grains (cereals) and tubers such as potato. It should be avoided by all blood groups. If raw starch is eaten, it will pass through the digestive tract until it reaches the lower part of the small intestine and into the large intestine (colon). There it is acted upon by some of the bacterial inhabitants which proliferate, causing a bacterial imbalance (dysbiosis) resulting in the production of large quantities of gas and irritants likely to cause painful intestinal spasms.

The Blood type groups
Features in common.

Cooked starch, on the other hand, is readily digested and converted rapidly into sugar. Any excess that cannot be burned up by physical activity results in raised blood sugar levels and the formation of fat and weight increase. There is also consequent interferance with lipid metabolism and the resultant danger of atheromatous deposits in the lining of the blood vessels; precursors of stroke and heart attack.

Salt: is generally a non-requirement, being adequately supplied in any diet with a sufficiency of animal protein. Exceptions occur commonly in blood group type A, or among true vegetarians whose diet consists entirely of vegetable matter lacking in sodium. In such cases, sea salt from clean waters, bringing with it a balance of other minerals, is preferable. Excess salt in the diet is, in many cases, associated with raised blood pressure and with the removal of calcium from bone (osteoporosis).

Exercise: a most important common requirement for all blood group types. Type O has the greatest need of all blood groups for regular vigorous exercise, but some form of regular physical activity is an absolute requirement for all. Exercise is the important non-nutritional factor known to normalise blood pressure and cholesterol balance.

Weight Regulation:
Weight gain : to avoid

All blood groups suffer weight gain:
- from diets which include sugar and grains, especially wheat.
- *regular frequent* intake of raw cabbage, which interferes with thyroid function, lowering the metabolic rate.
- lack of appropriate exercise.

In addition:

Blood group type O should avoid regular use of sweetcorn, kidney beans and lentils.

Blood group type A should avoid excess meat, dairy products and kidney and lima beans.

Blood group type B should avoid lentils, peanuts, sesame and buckwheat.

Blood group type AB should be cautious with kidney and lima beans, seeds, sweetcorn and buckwheat.

Weight loss : to promote

All blood groups need to maintain physical activity suitable to the type, but exercise alone in the absence of correct nutrition will not promote weight loss.

Blood group type O must place the emphasis on increased variety of leafy green vegetables, including marine plants, seafoods and offals.

Blood group type A should reduce grains and starches and increase variety of leafy green vegetables.

The Blood type groups
Features in common.

Blood group type B should avoid grains and pulses and stay with leafy green vegetables, offal and eggs.

Blood group type AB does best by avoiding grains, pulses and starches, putting emphasis on seafoods, leafy green vegetables, maritime and marine plants and fruit.

These are general rules which work. The body has a remarkable weight-balancing mechanism. Given the right conditions, once the optimum weight has been attained, it will be maintained without further problem.

There is, of course, always an exception. One knows of the person who eats like a gannet and remains bean-pole thin, while another has only to wave the proverbial oily rag under the nose to gain weight. There is something wrong in each case.

Just as one swallow does not make a summer, so the exception does not prove the rule.

Chapter 19

Guidelines

. . . on a lighter note
Good for you

The Japanese eat very little fat and suffer fewer heart attacks than the Aussies, British or Americans.

Mexicans eat a lot of fat and suffer fewer heart attacks than the Aussies, British or Americans.

Africans drink very little red wine and suffer fewer heart attacks than the Aussies, British or Americans.

The French and Italians drink large amounts of red wine and suffer fewer heart attacks than the Aussies, British or Americans.

Germans drink a lot of beer and eats lots of sausages and fats and suffer fewer heart attacks than the Aussies, British or Americans.

Medical conclusion

Eat and drink what you like.
Speaking English is apparently what kills you.

anon.

Cooking Guidelines
Utensils and Cooking Techniques

Utensils

Cookware can be of iron[1], cast iron, stainless steel, enamelled iron or steel, tinned copper, earthenware (pottery), ceramic or glass.

Under no circumstances use aluminium or teflon coated vessels or aluminium ("silver") foil for cooking food. Aluminium is a highly reactive, toxic metal which is easily dissolved by acids in foods – especially vegetables and fruits. Have you noticed how shiny-bright a previously dull-looking aluminium pan appears after cooking tomatoes?

The best use for aluminium saucepans and milk bottle tops was found during the Second World War when they were melted down and made into fighter planes – Hurricanes and Spitfires.

Non-stick[2] coatings tend to be porous and soon wear to reveal the underlying aluminium surfaces.

---

[1] *Exclusive use of iron vessels may lead to excessive iron intake – see section on minerals; iron. The coating materials are suspect – classified in the US as being carcinogenic – with possible links to fetal development problems.*
[2] *An exception is a newly-developed ceramic coating on cast iron with quite magical properties.*

Cooking Techniques

Boiling

With the exception of some root vegetables, such as beetroot for salads, Jerusalem artichoke, celeriac and other vegetables like globe artichoke, cardoon, beans in pod (young broad, French, runner), peas in pod (mangetout, sugar-snap) where losses are small, do not cook vegetables by boiling. Valuable nutrients including minerals, vitamins, as well as flavours are either destroyed or leached into the water which is usually thrown away. What remains has been denatured by the high temperature. For this reason, pressure cookers should not be used for cooking vegetables; they are better reserved for cooking bones from fish or meat to make wonderful bases for soups and stews.

When making vegetable soups and stews, the water should be brought up rapidly to boiling point (thus inhibiting any bacterial contamination) and then the temperature immediately lowered and maintained *below* boiling point, where the surface of the water is hardly moving. This method, known as *anhepsetal* cooking, retains much of the value and flavours while minimising the losses.

Frying

Depending on what is being cooked, this is not as evil a method as we have been led to believe. Meat and fish, so long as they are not coated in batter, flour or breadcrumbs, do not absorb fat when fried – in fact, in the case of some meats, fat is actually released.

Cooking Guidelines
Cooking Techniques

The case for starchy foods is quite different. An example: 4 ounces (115g.) of potato will, in energy terms provide about 80Kcal., while the same weight of potato chips (French fries, US) will furnish 330 Kcal. and a similar quantity of potato crisps (chips, US) contributes a whopping 530Kcal. – *all of which extra is fat!*

The kind of fat used for frying is important *(see box)*. Use only sufficient to cover the bottom of the pan and *do not allow it to smoke*. Any fat acts primarily as a conductor of heat to the food that is being cooked. It prevents charring (burning), provides texture and is a conveyor of flavours. **Do not re-use; once only should be the rule.**

Wok stir-frying is a misnomer. It should properly be called wok cooking as I am reliably informed by an expert[1]. The method is common in many Asian countries where fuel is scarce and cooking oils are expensive. It is perfectly acceptable for cooking most kinds of food.

Meticulous preparation is required. Items that need thorough cooking, such as certain roots and some kinds of meat may need cutting into match-thin strips, while others that cook more rapidly, various leaves and fish, into graded, larger pieces.

The thin metal of the steel wok heats up very rapidly, a minimum, say a teaspoonful (5ml) of oil is added and almost immediately the prepared foods thrown in and stirred. The high heat produces steam in a flash and the food cooks rapidly in its own juices – not fried.

The Western misconception arises from not understanding (as I did not) the principle of the method and the necessity (or unwillingness to take the time) for the careful preparation of the food beforehand.

When using this method, take care not to be leaning over the wok and inhaling the fumes. A very large number of women in Asian countries who use this way of cooking, suffer from severe lung problems resulting from the inhalation of oil vapours.

Ridged frying pans, which can produce charring, should be used with great care.

Deep Frying

Deep frying is a method which involves sealing and browning by immersing food into a bath of oil or fat heated to a *maximum* temperature of 170°C (335°F). If not avoided altogether, it should be reserved for occasional, infrequent use for the following reasons:

- the cooking temperatures are too high[2];
- most items cooked in this way are starches, e.g. potato chips, pastry, fritters, bread dough or meats and fish coated with batter, breadcrumbs etc.;
- starches cooked at high temperatures undergo a chemical change. The dark brown colouration is associated with a carcinogen, *acrylamide*. While infrequent consumption may not impose a risk, regular eating of deep-fried foods is dangerous;

---

[1] *I am grateful to Anne Hanson for enlightenment and careful explanation of this most important distinction.*

[2] *Many deep-fryers are fitted with a thermostat. If so, use it. If not buy and use a thermometer!*

Cooking Guidelines
Techniques and Culinary Fats

Culinary Fats

The safest fat to use for all purposes, whether raw for salads or for cooking, is virgin (cold-pressed) olive oil; preferably unfiltered. This fruit oil (avocado is another) is considered by some authorities to confer benefits which are absent in seed oils. Being mono-unsaturated, olive oil is certainly more stable and less liable to toxic degradation than the polyunsaturated seed oils such as those derived from sunflower, safflower and corn. Nevertheless, it is best kept sealed in dark containers away from heat. In cooking, provided it is not used smoking-hot, olive oil is very heat stable.

There are other fats that can be used safely for particular purposes. They are mostly saturated; beef dripping, clarified butter or ghee used in Indian cuisine, coconut oil, cocoa butter and the lard – partly unsaturated – from free-ranging pigs, goose fat. How can I say this? Saturated fats, we are told, are "bad". Not necessarily so. Essentially they are – unlike the seed oils – completely stable, not only in storage but also when heated. Used correctly they are safe. They should not be used to excess and – this applies to any fat – never re-used.

Some oils, walnut and sesame, for example are valued for the flavour they can impart to dishes. They are very delicate and should be kept sealed in dark containers in the refrigerator. They should *never* be used to cook food. If required in a hot dish they can be added to it after it has been cooked. The usual use for such oils is to add piquancy to salad dishes.

- the oils used are of the cheaper "pure" vegetable oils (unspecified, unholy mixtures) or vulnerable polyunsaturated oils such as sunflower seed or corn (maize);

- the quantity of oil used in deep fryers is such that people will not dispose of the oil after a single use. The accumulation of resulting *trans* fatty acids which increases with repeated use, together with other substances from burnt material – many of which are recognised to be carcinogenic – constitutes a real danger which filtering does not remove. (This same danger applies to the too-regular eating of foods from commercial fried-food shops and restaurants);

- starches which have absorbed and been coated by fats, impose a problem of digestion. Instead of being dealt with higher up in the small intestine, they are not released until the fat coating has been removed lower down, where starch-digesting enzymes are lacking. The result is fermentation by opportunistic bacteria and the production of irritant, toxic materials (with subsequent damage to the intestinal lining) and serious unbalancing of the intestinal flora on which so much of our well-being depends;

- the ease and quickness of this way of cooking appeals to hard-pressed mothers and as a result too many children are being fed regularly in this manner, eating the "wrong" foods which lack true nutritional value, are energy dense and predisposing the new generation to a host of avoidable ills.

Cooking Guidelines
Cooking Techniques – grilling, roasting and vegetables

Grilling

The "grill" on domestic cookers, which delivers radiant heat from above the food, is technically a salamander – not a grill. Provided that it is used correctly so that the food being cooked is not burnt, it is perfectly acceptable.

Char-grilling and barbecue, unless very carefully controlled, are not to be recommended. Too often, the meat or fish is charred (hence the name) i.e. burnt, with the production of dangerous chemicals in the blackened portions. These are capable of producing cancer, principally of the stomach among those individuals whose production of gastric hydrochloric acid is insufficient or absent.

Roasting – oven cooking

Meat, fish, root vegetables and tubers can be cooked in this way, as can many other vegetables including aubergine, capsicums (sweet peppers), onions, celery, chicory, fennel, marrow and squash: smeared with olive oil and seasoned with herbs. Meat should be raised from the bottom of the baking dish to allow excess fat to drain away. Fish may be laid on the bottom of the dish, so allowing it to be cooked in its own juice.

The trick to roasting is to put the meat or fish in a very hot oven for a short time (15-30 minutes). This allows surface coagulation, so "sealing" the contained juices. The temperature should then be reduced, allowing heat to penetrate and cooking to proceed.

Do not overcook meat or fish in this fashion.

Cooking vegetables

Apart from my comments about boiling, most vegetables can be cooked by steaming, so retaining valuable nutrients. Sautéeing in the French manner is also a good method: freshly washed leafy vegetables are put into a dry pan with a little olive oil, a pinch of sea-salt and covered with a tight lid. Put the pan on to high heat for two minutes, give the pan a good shake (holding the lid down!) and put the pan back on low heat and allow the contents to simmer gently. Microwave cooking of vegetables has become a popular way of cooking vegetables. It is very quick, economic of energy and minimises the loss of nutrient content. On the other hand, I know several researchers in the field of nutrition who will not stay in the same room when the microwave cooker is operating because of the secondary, harmonic electromagnetic radiation that is present. They claim that it is harmful.

Mushrooms

Although this is not meant to be a cookery book, I feel that it is important to mention this particular, valuable – in Britain, rather feared – food.

All *edible* mushrooms and fungi (cultivated or wild) may be used. They may be braised in similar manner to other vegetables; fried, roasted or added to other dishes such as soups and stews. Some can be eaten raw in salads, others dried and stored.

When using wild mushrooms or fungi, make sure that you have identified them correctly *before* cooking and eating. Mistakes cannot be rectified later!

Guidelines

Quantities

Over many thousands of years, Man has had to adapt to fluctuations, sometimes extreme, in availability of foods; feast and famine. Those people with the resilience to cope are our ancestors; survival of the fittest.

Currently our lives are more directed by the clock than by our instincts: 8am, breakfast; 1 o'clock, lunch; 4 o'clock, tea; 8 o'clock, dinner; regardless of appetite or need. Regularity has become the norm and, sometimes, obsessive rigidity.

Re-introducing flexibility is important for our physical *and mental* health. The occasional one-day fast (but no longer than that), or the meat-free day, does no harm at all; in many cases is beneficial.

Here and there in this book, I have mentioned "daily requirements" in relation to proteins, vitamins, minerals and others. These figures have been derived from many years of observation, research and, not infrequently, guesswork. They do not in fact specify a *must* for every single day but more truly the *average* requirement.

The challenges provided by fluctuations, whether of climate, weather, food types and amount – even infection or injury – provide the stimuli that prompt resilience, the ability to "bounce back" which is, after all, a mark of health.

Quantity – How much?

Protein

Question How much meat or fish should I eat in a day?

Answer In the UK the official figure for the average daily requirement is *70 grams*.

As protein constitutes only one fifth of the total weight of meat or fish, this would be equivalent to 350g (12 ounces - $^3/_4$lb) of either. If, as some authorities believe, the amount of protein should be 100g, the equivalent amount would be 500g (17 $^1/_2$ ounces - slightly over 1lb).

In fact you would not require even these amounts, bearing in mind that a significant part of the food should consist of vegetables in variety. These contain the amino acids necessary to build new proteins.

Here is a simple rule of thumb method which enables you judge the amount of fish or meat you need in a day. It works well in practice, so throw away your slide-rule and letter balance:

A piece of meat or fish, the size of your hand, including fingers and thumb and 19mm ($^3/_4$ inches) thick, depending on how big are your hands, would weigh anything between 360 and 440 g (12$^1/_2$ - 15 ounces or about $^3/_4$ - 1lb) and supply between 70 and 90g of protein. Similarly, a piece the size of the palm of your hand of similar thickness would weigh somewhere between 270 and 330g (9 - 11$^1/_2$ ounces or $^1/_2$ – $^3/_4$ lb) and provide between 54 and 66 g of protein. These figures would correspond to the contribution made by four to six 60 g (2$^1/_2$ ounces) eggs from free-ranging hens. So, don't fuss over precise amounts. You don't have to be more accurate than this.

Guidelines

Quantities

Question As a complete vegetarian (vegan), how can I obtain sufficient protein?

Answer All plants supply amino acids from which the body can build its protein. Individual vegetables do not supply the full range that we need so that it is necessary to make sure of a mixture of different vegetables during the course of the day, although not necessarily at the same meal. Mushrooms and fungi are good sources of protein and of an amino acid, lysine, which is often lacking in plants. Legumes – dried beans, peas and lentils – are rich in amino acids and, together with other vegetables, are good providers of protein. Soya beans can supply the full range of amino acids.

Take Note:

100 g of *dried* legumes can be considered to be approximately equal in protein content to the same weight of meat or fish. 100 g of *cooked* legumes, because of the absorption of water, will provide *only one quarter* of the amount of protein.

Fat

There is a general acceptance among experts that, ideally, our daily intake of fat should contribute between 25% and 30% of our total energy requirement. For a relatively sedentary person whose daily energy expenditure is 2,000 Kcals, this would amount to a contribution from fat of between 500 and 600 Kcals. Fat has an energy value of 9 Kcals per gram (see section on Fats) so that the actual quantity would lie between 55 and 60 g (2-2½ounces).

For a more active person expending up to 2,500 Kcals daily, the requirement from fat would be between 625 and 750 Kcals, equivalent to 70 and 80 g fat.

In household terms:

60 g of olive oil would equal 6 tablespoons (180ml);

60 g of solid fat, e.g. beef dripping, 2 rounded tablespoonsful;

80 g of olive oil would equal 8 tablespoonsful (250ml);

80 g of solid fat, about 2½ tablespoonsful.

Some fat would be naturally in the food, some used in cooking and some added; as in salad dressings and mayonnaise.

Much conflicting information concerning fat in the diet has confused and alarmed many people, leading them to become fearful – even paranoid – about fat, regarding it as an evil, not a necessity. This mistake has led them to avoid even the oily fish, believing them (wrongly) to be fattening and not realising that the essential fatty acids present are vital to health; the structural fats used for repair and maintenance, not for fuel or for creating fatty tissue.

It is just as important, therefore, not to have too little fat in the diet (going below 20% can involve a risk to health) as it is not to have too much.

Guidelines
Quantities

Carbohydrates

Carbohydrates are essentially fuel. If we are eating correctly, they should provide 50% or more of our energy needs. Carbohydrates have no specific body-building qualities[1]. There are three main categories:

1. Simple carbohydrates; sugars such as glucose, fructose and dextrose (table sugar). There are two groups:

    intrinsic, found in fruits and certain vegetables, such as carrots. They are incorporated into the plant structure and released relatively slowly;

    extrinsic, have been extracted from their sources and include table sugar, syrups, treacles and honey. They are often added to other foods including confectioneries and soft drinks;

2. Starches, sometimes called (wrongly, I think) complex carbohydrates and consisting of groups of sugar molecules (see section Components of food – carbohydrates *p80&81*). They exist in all grains, most roots and tubers (e.g. potato) but not in fruits except bananas. Cooked – not raw – starch is very rapidly broken down during digestion to form sugars;

3. Truly complex carbohydrates are to be found in all fresh leafy green vegetables and some tubers such as Jerusalem artichokes and water chestnuts. They consist of polysaccharides and oligosaccharides, which are digested very much more slowly. Some oligosaccharides, inulin and oligofructose which we cannot digest, are necessary for the growth of beneficial bacteria – the bowel flora – of the digestive tract.

A fourth category, the carbohydrates contributed by meat or fish can for practical purposes, be ignored if these items are not being eaten in excess. Their contributions tend to be in the form of oligosaccharides and muco-polysaccharides.

How much

Starches and sugars are energy-dense and must be regarded with great caution, used sparingly or even avoided totally. They supply ready fuel very quickly, causing a rapid rise in blood sugar levels and subsequently an increase in circulating triglyceride fats. Because they lack bulk, these carbohydrates rarely provide a sense of repletion unless eaten to excess (except when accompanied by fat and so increasingly the energy content). The likely consequence is weight increase, leading to obesity and all the attendant dangers.

---

[1] All carbohydrates are reduced by digestion to various simple sugars. Thus none can be considered as being specific for building any particular component or tissue.
The body is, however, a fantastic chemical workshop and from the simple sugars derived from food, manufactures new sugars of numbers, size and complexity only now being discovered. The range extends even further than that presently known for proteins and encompasses the structure and function of every tissue. This newly-discovered internal magic will reveal eventually much more information about how our bodies function.
It does **not** alter any of the rules already outlined for eating correctly.

Guidelines
Quantities and The Glycaemic Index

Carbohydrates from fresh leafy vegetables are less concentrated and of a different nature. They are accompanied by phyto (plant) chemicals and consequently are absorbed more slowly and over a longer time, so avoiding the precipitate rise in blood sugar and the interference with the blood lipids. The lower energy content means that much larger quantities of vegetables can safely be consumed, together with all their other valuable nutrients, so providing the comfort and satisfaction of repletion without danger. In other words, vegetables can be consumed freely; they provide their own safe limit.

Sugars in fruits are released relatively slowly and, in this regard considered to be "safe", but with a caveat. Remember that fruits lack the body-building materials present in vegetables and so should take second place. *They should not be consumed without limit or instead of vegetables.*

The Glycaemic Index

Carbohydrates and carbohydrate-containing foods that form part of today's diet vary considerably in their effect on our health. It makes sense, therefore, to have a means of distinguishing those which are valuable and those which are harmful. Whatever your aim – to maintain or improve your health, lose weight, avoid the consequences of, or improve your chances against such illnesses as heart disease, arthritis, diabetes or obesity – the Glycaemic Index is your tool. Although only an approximation, it is sufficiently accurate to provide a very good, practical working guide. The lists in the following tables will help you – here is where you can use your imagination.

If you are young, fit of normal weight and active, it may be possible for you to stray from list A-B, C – even D, occasionally. If you are not so young or fit, are overweight and less active, to do so would put you at risk. So, stick to the guidelines.

A Good or Favourable Carbohydrates (15 or less) Eat freely

Leafy green vegetables: some examples;

Artichoke (globe), asparagus, green beans in pod (young broad beans, dwarf French, pole and runner), leaf beet (chard), broccoli, burnet, brussels sprouts, cabbage, calaloo, cardoon, cauliflower, celery, chicories (endives), corn salad (mache, lambs' lettuce), claytonia (winter purslane, miner's lettuce), mustard, onion, parsley, peas in pod (mangetout, sugar snap), purslane, rocket (roquette, rucola), sea kale, shallot, sorrel, spinach, New Zealand spinach, watercress.

Roots and tubers: Artichokes (Jerusalem), celeriac, ginger, mangel, parsnip. radishes, salsify, scorzonera, swede, turnip, water chestnuts;

Fruits include: Apple*, apricot*, blackberry, black (and red and white) currant, blueberry, cape gooseberry (chinese lantern, physalis edulis), chinese gooseberry (Kiwi fruit, achtinidia chinensis), cranberry, cherry, elderberry, fig,* gooseberry, grapefruit, grape*, lemon, lime,

Guidelines
The Glycaemic Index

mango, medlar, mulberry, nectarine, orange, passion fruit, peach, pear, plum*, quince, raspberry, strawberry, tangerine, New Zealand tree tomato.

*often preserved by drying.

"Fruits" regarded as vegetables: Aubergine, avocado, capsicums (sweet peppers), courgette, cucumber, okra (bhindi, ladies' fingers), peppers (chilli), tomatillo (physalis exocarpa), tomato.

Edible fungi: Include a very wide range of wild and cultivated mushrooms, toadstools and truffles.

Nuts: Almond, filberts (cob or hazel), pecan, pine, pistachios and walnuts;

Seeds: include caraway, poppy, pumpkin, sesame and sunflower.

B Moderate Carbohydrates (15 – 35) Eat occasionally

Roots and tubers: carrots, new potatoes, sweet potatoes, beetroots;

Pulses (legumes): dried broad beans (fava), other various dried beans, peas, lentils, chickpeas, "monkey nut" (peanuts);

Fruits: citrus (oranges, clementines, grapefruit), grapes, mangos, papayas;

Nuts: Brazil, cashew, chestnut, macadamia, coconut;

Chocolate: 70% or more cocoa solids (energy dense because of the fat content);

C Borderline (40 – 60) Treat with caution: little and seldom

Fruits: bananas, dates, melon, pineapple

Dried fruits:

Sweet corn:

Burghl: (cracked wheat) and other cracked (not ground) grains.

D Bad (60 – 100) Treat as potentially dangerous: avoid altogether where possible by anyone at risk.

Sugars: glucose, sucrose (table sugar) white or brown, honey, syrups, soft drinks, snack bars. Although fructose has a low GI (20) it is in quantity dangerous and should, therefore, be avoided except where it occurs naturally in fruits (see section of Food – sugar, page 53-57);

Fruits: melons, pumpkins;

Roots and tubers: potatoes in all forms – baked, boiled, chipped, crisped, fried or roasted;

Grains: Barley, buckwheat*, maize, millet, oats, quinoa*, rice, rye, wheat, wild rice.

* not members of the grass family; graminae.

Cereals: all cereals – refined or wholemeal – breads, breakfast cereals, cakes+, croissants+, pastas, pastries+, short breads+.

N.B. Cracked grains have a slightly lower GI than milled grains because they are less easily digested. The finer the milling and the longer the cooking, the higher the GI (and the danger).

+ Apart from having a high GI, these items are more energy dense because of the fat content.

Nutrition for the Family

The older man and woman

copy of a letter sent to the Daily Mail by a grateful patient of mine

> **Your article re. "The Stone Age Diet".**
>
> 2 years ago, at the Royal Brompton Chest Hospital after an extensive 10 days of tests including allergy testing I was diagnosed with emphysema. I was put on a number of turbo inhalers, pills and a nebuliser inhaler of pure Salbutamol and Pulmacort.
>
> I could not walk 10 yards without fighting for my breath and after any exertion I would suffer chronic asthma attacks. Life was intolerable and as a very active person I was reduced to a complete invalid.
>
> My daughter works for a New York doctor who with his family flies the Atlantic to visit a doctor in Harley St whom they swear by. He is a diagnostician, consultant and homoepath and my daughter insisted that I go and see him as I had nothing to lose and everything to gain.
>
> I parked my car at the northern end of Harley St. and had to walk the entire length, as his consulting rooms were at the other end. I had to stop six times after walking a few yards to fight for my breath.
>
> After an hour's consultation with him he sent me for a series of blood tests. When he had the results I went for second visit to him for his diagnosis. With a number of vitamin/mineral supplements, I was put on a diet of non dairy, non wheat including pasta, no sugar no bananas or dates, no honey with the instructions "think prehistoric". Plenty of green vegetables meat fish and fruit.
>
> A copy of his diet is attached, He also said that he would have me walking round a golf course, to which my reply was "And pigs will fly".
>
> This visit to the doctor was in September 2002 and on the 19th December 2002 I walked 18 holes around Ruislip golf course and this year, at the age of 73, I have given up on a lot of my puffers and feel 200% better.
>
> So your article on the "Stone Age Diet" really hit a chord with me and I felt that I had to write to you of my success and new lease of life, all due to a doctor I call a miracle maker.
>
> Alan Gilbey

Chapter 20

Postscript

Postscript

I could have written the principles of Healthy Eating on the back of an envelope or a postcard, so – instead of writing an entire book – why didn't I?

People today need reasons for what they do. Wherever you and I may have been born or raised, we have acquired ideas of what is "normal" eating, together with attendant habits and prejudices. To alter them (particularly the last), we need to know the what and to understand the why. Today, that knowledge exists – millions of man-years of it – of what constitutes good food and how it can be produced.

Our pre-agricultural ancestors did not need this knowledge, surrounded as they were by foods to which their bodies were attuned: leafy vegetables in abundant variety, tubers, fruits, fish, lean meats and the right kinds of fats; but no starches and minimal sugar. Despite many adaptive changes we still retain the body chemistry of our ancestors, but our food has strayed wildly off course; principally with the excessive introduction of sugars and starches – previously absent and for which we are ill-equipped.

Certainly, agriculture as we know it today has to be turned on its head! (see chapter: Agriculture is not natural). Such a change cannot be accomplished overnight; it will take decades, *starting now*. Neither should it be left entirely to national governments to accomplish. A global effort is necessary, combining the knowledge of anthropologists, archeologists, agronomists, climatologists as well as experts in geology, marine and animal husbandry, human and veterinary medicine, plus the determination and perseverance of people like you and me to see it through. The resultant transformation would not only ensure sufficient food for the rising numbers of people while preserving the animal populations – with adequate room for both – but would enhance the environment, rather than destroy it.

Nor do we have to wait for tomorrow to adopt the ancestral way of eating. We can do it now. In the developed countries, the right foods are readily available. Make your choice. Elsewhere, with few exceptions, foods indigenous to the area, climate and season can be grown best suited to the needs of the local people. A bonus would be a reduction in the colossal cost and waste of resources arising from the current fashion of transporting large amounts of (often unsuitable) foods thousands of miles across the world.

So . . . no envelope, no postcard; only a book.

Dear Reader, I wish you well.

A.S.

Be careful about reading health books. You may die of a misprint.

Mark Twain

Bibliography and References

Some of the references given below, dating back a century or more, may seem to be irrelevant to today's needs – not "up-to-date". The fact is that Truth does not alter with time.

Older books are not always easily obtainable, although many have been reprinted. Many can also be obtained from the local library today through inter-library loan.

Origins/Evolution

References:

The Ancestor's Tale A Pilgrimage to the Dawn of Life Richard Dawkins pub. Weidenfeld & Nicolson, London ISBN 0 297 82503 8

Yudkin J. **Archeology and the nutritionist** (in Ucko PJ and Dimbley EW, Eds) **The domestication and exploitation of plants and animals.** Chicago Aldine 1969.

Trowell HG and Burkitt DP, Eds **Western diseases, their emergence and prevention.** Harvard University Press 1981.

Crawford M.A. **Fatty acid ratios in free-living and domestic animals.** Lancet 1968.

Crawford M.A., Gale MM, Woodford MH. **Linoleic acid and linolenic acid on elongation products in muscle tissue of** *cyncerus caffer* **and other various ruminant species.** J. Biochem 1969.

Crawford M.A., Gale MM, Woodford MH. **Muscle and adipose tissue lipids of the wart-hog** *Phaecohoerus arthiopicus*. Int. J. Biochem 1970.

Agriculture

Titles:

The Living Soil Lady Eve Balfour pub. Faber and Faber 1950

The Way of the Land Sir George Stapledon pub. Faber and Faber 1943

Prophet of the New Age, The Life and Thoughts of Sir George Stapledon FRS Robert Waller pub. Faber and Faber 1962

Tree Crops A permanent Agriculture Professor J. Russell Smith pub. The Devin-Adair Company.

Forest Farming J. Sholto Douglas and Robert A de J Hart pub. Watkins London. ISBN 0-7224-0842-6

Grass Farming/Grassland Management André Voisin and many other titles *note seek publishers (Anglo/French) & ISBN*

Rotation Grazing: The Meeting of Cows and Grass: A manual of Grass Productivity André Voisin with A. Lecomte pub. Crosby Lockwood, 1962

also by André Voisin:

Soil Grass and Cancer Paris 1969

Grass Productivity 1958

Grass Tetany 1963 and many others

Chisel Ploughing seek author (Australian) pub? ISBN

The Forest Garden Robert Hart ISBN 0-948826-19-3

The Parable of Green Mountain David Wilkinson Journal of Biogeography, vol. 31 (2004).

Bibliography and references

Nutrition and Health

Titles:
The Work of Sir Robert McCarrison edited by H.M. Sinclair
pub. Faber and Faber 1953
Nutrition and Health Sir Robert McCarrison 1944
(originally Nutrition and National Health 1936) Faber and Faber.
Re-published 1982 by McCarrison Society ISBN 0-946153-00-0
What we eat today Michael and Sheilagh Crawford pub. Neville Spearman
ISBN 0-85435-360-7
Soil Food and Health in a Changing World Contributions from many distinguished scientists, doctors and authors.
pub. AB Academic Publishers ISBN 0-907360-00-9
This Slimming Business 1958, The Slimmers Cookbook 1961, The Complete Slimmer 1964, Pure White and Deadly 1972, This Nutrition Business 1976 (ISBN 0-7067-0185-2) Professor John Yudkin pub. Denis Poynter.
Nutrition and Physical Degeneration Weston A. Price DDS
pub. Price-Pottenger Foundation. ISBN 0-916-764-00-1 www.ppnf.org
Expanded edition 1980 ISBN 978-0-916764-20-3
Biochemical Individuality Dr Roger A. Williams pub. University of Texas 1956

Fibre

Titles:
The Saccharine Disease T.L. Cleave, MRCP
pub. John Wright and Sons Ltd. ISBN 0-7236-0368-5
Diabetes, Coronary Thrombosis and the Saccharine Disease
T.L. Cleave and T.D. Campbell pub. John Wright and Sons Ltd
Don't forget the fibre in your diet Denis Burkitt MD FRCS FRS.
pub. Martin Dunitz   ISBN 09063-348-06-4
                     ISBN 09063-348-07-2
The Lactic Acid Bacteria and their Role in Human Health
Dr Nigel Plummer BSc PhD

Lipids

References:
Professor Hugh Sinclair
Preventions of coronary heart disease: the role of essential fatty acids.
Postgraduate Medical Journal (August 1980)

Bibliography and references

Lipids continued

References:

Stress and Hypertension: Dietary and Metabolic Factors in the Development of Atherosclerosis.

Contributions to Nephrology Vol 30 (Kerger, Bosch 1982).

Essential Fatty Acids and Chronic Degenerative Diseases from Nutrition and Killer diseases:

The effects of dietary factors on fatal chronic diseases. Ed. J. Rose New Jersey: Noyes Publ. 1982.

Professor Michael Crawford

The Driving force: Food, Evolution and the Future (1989) – another classic
Evidence for the unique function of DNA during the evolution of the modern hominid brain.
In conjunction with Bloom M., Broadhurst C.L. et al. (1999)

Dietary fats and fatty acids in human health care Plummer Nigel, PhD. pub. Bio Med Publications Ltd, Harbourne, BIRMINGHAM B32 2HR UK

The Food and Agriculture Organisation of the United Nations Dietary Fats and Oils in human nutrition ISBN 92-5-100802-7

Fats that Heal Fats that Kill Erasmus, Udo PhD pub. Alive Books, B.C.
ISBN 0-920470-40-8
ISBN 0-920470-38-6

Allergy

Titles:

An Alternative Approach to Allergies Theron G. Randolph MD and Ralph W. Moss MD. pub. Lippincot and Crowell ISBN 0-0690-01998-x

Food Allergy and Intolerance Professor Jonathan Brostoff and Dr Stephen J. Challacombe pub. Bailliére and Tindal ISBN 0-7020-1156-8

Food and Society

Titles:

Technological Eating Magnus Pyke
ISBN 0-7195-2576-4

Food and Society Magnus Pyke
ISBN 0-7195-1801-6

and numerous others pub. John Murray

Bibliography and references

Therapy through Nutrition

Titles:
The Healing Nutrients Within Eric Bravermann MD and Carl C. Ppfeiffer MD
pub. Keats publishing Inc. ISBN 087983-384-X

Mental and Elemental Nutrients Carl C. Pfeiffer MD pub. Keats Publishing Inc.
ISBN 0-87983-114-6

How to Live with Schizophrenia Abram Hoffer MD and Humphrey Osmond MD
pub. Citadel Press ISBN 0-8065-0665-2

Nutrition Against Disease Dr Roger A. Williams
pub. Bantam Books ISBN 0-553-20086-0

Nutritional Medicine Dr Stephen Davies and Dr Alan Stewart
pub. Accelerated Learning Systems ISBN 0-905553-63-2

Sauvez Votre Corps Dr Catharine Kousemine
pub. J'ai Lu Editions Robert Laffont, S.A. ISBN 2-277-07029-7

Nutrition for the Family

Title:
Brain Child Tony Buzan pub. Thorsons ISBN 00-00-716607-9
Tony Buzan is an internationally recognised and acclaimed educationalist. His book deals less with food for the body as with nurture of the whole person. It seems that the more that countries "develop" the more is the family threatened with disintegration. If Mankind is to survive, the integrity of the family, its safety and of every individual in it, is paramount.
This book is a must for all parents and parents-to-be; also for all school children from their early 'teens until they leave school.

Genetics

Title:
Your Family Tree Connection Dr Chris Reading and Ross C. Meillon
pub. Keats Publishing Inc. ISBN 0-07983-483-6

Remedial Dentistry – Mercury

Title:
Menace in the Mouth? Dr Jack Levenson
pub. Brompton Health ISBN 0-9534734-3-0

Bibliography and references

Blood Groups

Titles:
Eat right 4 your type Peter J. D'Adamo pub. Century London
ISBN 0-9063-348-06-4
ISBN 0-9063-348-07-2
Blood Relations: Blood Groups and Anthropology Mourant A.E. pub. Oxford University Press 1984
Blood Groups in Man Race R.R. and Sanger R. pub. Blackwell Scientific 1975

Exercise

Title:
The New Power Program Michael Colgan PhD., pub. Apple Publishing Co. Ltd., Vancouver, Canada. ISBN 1-896817-00-9.
Dr Colgan, a competent biochemist, is a world leader in the field of physical education and training. This book is written for professionals (it is **not** a "do-it-yourself" work), but nevertheless valuable to anyone genuinely interested in physical development. It describes in detail methods of exercise and the rationale for the enhancement of the body/musculature and its adaptation in different pursuits. I do **not**, however, advocate anyone's following the nutritional advice – especially the use of specially formulated drinks (designed for the "bigger-is-better" market) without proper professional advice.

Useful publications

Titles:
Nutrition and Health a quarterly journal with a distinguished international editorial board, ISSN 0260-1060 Pub. AB Academic Publishers, PO Box 97, Berkhamstead, Hertfordshire HP4 2PX UK
Living Earth a quarterly journal published by the Soil Association ISSN 1360-1741

Useful Organisations

The International Society for Prenatal and Perinatal Psychology and Medicine, Heidelberg, Germany.
The McCarrison Society Chairman: Professor Michael A. Crawford
Institute of Brain Chemistry and Human Nutrition,
London Metropolitan University, North London Campus, 166-222 Holloway Road, LONDON N7 8DB UK

Bibliography and references

Useful Organisations continued
Organic Agriculture

The Soil Association Chairman: Craig Sams, Director: Patrick Holden
Bristol House, 40-56 Victoria Street, BRISTOL BS1 6BY UK

Elm Farm Research Centre Director Lawrence Woodward, OBE, Hamstead Marshall, near NEWBURY, Berkshire RG20 0HR UK

Sheepdrove Organic Farm Founders and Owners: Peter and Juliet Kindersley, Warren Farm, LAMBOURN, Berkshire RG17 7UU UK

Faculty for Biological Agriculture Sciences Kassel University, 37213 Witzenhausen, Germany

Federal Agency for Nature Conservation *Bundesamt für Naturschutz*, President: Professor Dr Hartmut Vogtmann, Konstantin Strasse 110, 53179 Bonn, Germany

Canadian Organic Growers 323 Chapel Street, Ottowa, Ontario, KIN 722 Canada.

Foresight Association for the Promotion of Pre-Conceptual Care
Founder: Mrs Peter Barnes,
Foresight, 178 Hawthorn Road, Bognor Regis, PO21 2UY UK

Facilities

Biolab Medical Unit Directors: Dr Stephen Davies and Dr Nicholas Miller for analyses through hair, sweat, blood and urine of minerals, vitamins, essential fatty acids, cholesterolesters and specific hormonal and bio functional assays.
9 Weymouth Street, LONDON W1 UK